# Essential Sports Medicine

# Essential Sports Medicine

Joseph E. Herrera
Editor
Department of Rehabilitation Medicine,
Interventional Spine and Sports, Mount Sinai Medical Center
New York, NY

Grant Cooper
Editor
New York Presbyterian Hospital
New York, NY

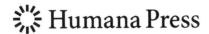 Humana Press

*Editors*
Joseph E. Herrera
Department of Rehabilitation Medicine
Interventional Spine & Sports
Mount Sinai Medical Center
New York, NY

Grant Cooper
New York Presbyterian Hospital
New York, NY


*Series Editors*
Joseph E. Herrera
Department of Rehabilitation Medicine
Interventional Spine and Sports
Mount Sinai Medical Center
New York, NY

Grant Cooper
New York Presbyterian Hospital
New York, NY

ISBN: 978-1-58829-985-7          e-ISBN: 978-1-59745-414-8
DOI: 10.1007/978-1-59745-414-8

Library of Congress Control Number

*Cover illustration*:

Printed on acid-free paper

9 8 7 6 5 4 3 2 1

springer.com

# Preface

Sports medicine is a popular medical subspecialty. Several types of medical specialists participate, to a varying extent, in the care of sports medicine complaints. These include family practitioners, internists, physiatrists, orthopedists, neurologists, emergency room doctors, and neurosurgeons. While some doctors undergo formal training in a sports medicine fellowship, others simply try to adapt their musculoskeletal medicine training (which in some fields may be limited) to the care of patients with sports injuries.

Sports medicine certainly overlaps with general musculoskeletal medicine, but there are important differences of which to be aware. *Essential Sports Medicine* was created with this in mind. We believe that *Essential Sports Medicine* provides the highest yield, comprehensive, pertinent information about sports medicine so that the busy clinician can find it accessible and practical. We hope that medical students, residents, and fellows will also find *Essential Sports Medicine* useful for providing an accessible overview of the most salient points in the field of sports medicine.

As editors, we were fortunate to find many expert physicians ready and willing to contribute to this project. This book reflects their commitment to their work, and their dedication to teaching and their patients. We hope you find it as interesting and enjoyable to read as it was for us to create.

*Joseph E. Herrera*
*Grant Cooper*

# Acknowledgments

JH: First I would like to thank my friend and co-editor, Dr. Grant Cooper. Without his endless patience, professionalism, and energy, the completion of this book would not have been possible. I would like to extend my great appreciation to all of the expert authors who have taken time out of their very busy schedules to give their invaluable contributions to this book. A special thanks to Dr. Barry Jordan, Dr. Robert Gotlin, Dr. Stuart Kahn, Dr. Alex Lee, Dr. Lisa Bartoli, Dr. Gregory Mulford, and Dr. Kristjan Ragnarsson, who have made me into the physician I am today through their example and leadership.

I would also like to thank Dr. Ana Bracilovic and Dr. Zinovy Meyler for staying late and being patient while we achieved the ideal photographs for the book. Lastly, my gratitude to Humana–Springer, especially Richard Lansing, Editor, for giving us the opportunity to write and publish this book and our book series.

GC: This book has been collaborative effort in every sense. As such, there are many people to thank. Thank you first to my co-editor, colleague, and good friend Dr. Joe Herrera. I could not ask for a better person with whom to work. Of course this book would not have been possible without the selfless dedication of the many expert authors who gave their time, energy, and expertise to making it as good as it is, and I extend my gratitude to each of them.

Thank you to my wife, Dr. Ana Bracilovic, and to Dr. Zinovy Meyler for serving as the models for the pictures in this book.

Thank you also to my many mentors for teaching, inspiring and encouraging me each step of the way. In particular, thank you to Dr. Robert Gotlin, Dr. Stuart Kahn, Dr. Alex Lee, Dr. Gregory Lutz, Dr. Paul Cooke, and Dr. Richard Meyer.

I would like to extend a special thank you to Richard Lansing, our editor at Humana–Springer. He has been a true professional in every sense of the word.

# Contents

# Contributors

Lisa Bartoli, DO
Team Physician, Women's USA Rugby, The Continuum Center
for Health and Healing, Beth Israel Medical Center, New York, NY

Thomas N. Bryce, MD
Department of Rehabilitation Medicine, The Mount Sinai Medical Center,
New York, NY

Grant Cooper, MD
Sports, Spine, and Musculoskeletal Rehabilitation, Beth Israel Medical Center,
New York, NY

Michael Dambeck, DO
Department of Rehabilitation Medicine, The Mount Sinai Medical Center,
New York, NY

Marc Effron, MD
New York-Presbyterian Hospital, The University Hospital of Columbia
and Cornell, New York, NY

Stephen Gelfman, DDS, MD
Surgery Oral and Maxillofacial, Long Island Jewish Medical Center,
New York, NY

Robert S. Gotlin, DO
Orthopedic and Sports Rehabilitation, Beth Israel Medical Center, New York, NY

Joseph E. Herrera, DO
Interventional Spine and Sports Medicine Division, Department of
Rehabilitation Medicine, Mount Sinai School of Medicine,
New York, NY

Victor Ibrahim, MD
Department of Rehabilitation Medicine, New York-Presbyterian Hospital,
The University Hospital of Columbia and Cornell, New York, NY

Barry D. Jordan, MD, MPH
Brain Injury Program, Burke Rehabilitation Hospital, White Plains, New York,
Chief Medical Officer, New York State Athletic Commission
New York, NY

Dov Kolker, MD
Department of Orthopaedics, Mount Sinai School of Medicine, New York, NY

Jennifer Kurz, MD
Department of Physical Medicine and Rehabilitation, Mount Sinai School
of Medicine, New York, NY

Aaron M. Levine, MD
New York-Presbyterian Hospital, The University Hospital of Columbia
and Cornell, New York, NY

Daniel Leung, DO
Department of Rehabilitation Medicine, The Mount Sinai Medical Center,
New York, NY

Gregory E. Lutz, MD
Physiatrist-in-Chief, Hospital for Special Surgery, Clinical
Rehabilitation Medicine, New York-Presbyterian Hospital, New York, NY

Jeffrey I. Mechanick, MD, FACP, FACE, FACN
Department of Endocrinology, Director, Metabolic Support Service, Mount Sinai
School of Medicine, New York, NY

Dorothy A. Miller, MD
Spinal Cord Injury Rehabilitation, The Mount Sinai Medical Center,
New York, NY

Necolle Morgado, DO
Department of Physical Medicine and Rehabilitation, The Mount Sinai Medical
Center, New York, NY

Danielle Marie Perret, MD
Department of Rehabilitation Medicine, Mount Sinai School of Medicine,
The Mount Sinai Medical Center, New York, NY

Parag Sheth, MD
Department of Rehabilitation Medicine, Mount Sinai School of Medicine,
New York, NY

Earl L. Smith, MD., PhD
Department of Rehabilitation Medicine, Mount Sinai School of Medicine,
New York, New York

Fani Thomson, DO
Department of Rehabilitation Medicine, Mount Sinai School of Medicine,
New York, NY

Elise Weiss, MD
Clinical Instructor, Physical Medicine and Rehabilitation, New York-Presbyterian
Hospital at Weill Cornell, New York, NY

# Chapter 1
# Preparticipation Evaluation

**Jennifer Kurz, Joseph E. Herrera, and Robert S. Gotlin**

## 1   Introduction

The preparticipation evaluation (PPE) is a medical assessment of athletes performed prior to their participation in various types and levels of sports. It encompasses obtaining the athlete's medical history, performing a physical examination, and very importantly, identifying pertinent risk factors potentially prohibiting the athlete from sports participation, all of which guide the physician in making decisions about an athlete's safe participation in sports. There are three basic outcomes of the PPE: full clearance—without restriction, limited clearance, or no clearance. The decision about clearance is multifactorial and must be done with the best interest of the athlete in mind. The physician must be familiar with the basic category of sport in which the athlete is involved, whether it is a contact or collision sport, limited contact/collision sport, or a noncontact sport. Noncontact sports can be further characterized by their strenuousness.

## 2   Goals of a Preparticipation Evaluation

1. Ensure the player's safety.
2. Determine the player's individual level of fitness and health.
3. Ascertain the player's physical maturity and cardiovascular fitness, and identify pre-existing injuries and other pertinent medical conditions.
4. Document all risk factors, including family history, which may necessitate restriction of the athlete's participation in a particular sport.
5. Counsel the patient on various health risk behaviors and other health-related issues that may arise.

J.E. Herrera and G. Cooper (eds.), *Essential Sports Medicine*,
doi: 10.1007/978-1-59745-414-8, © Humana Press 2008

## 3   Timing of Preparticipation Evaluations

The frequency and timing of preparticipation evaluations vary slightly from state to state, but in general they are done annually. All states, including the District of Columbia, require physical exams prior to high school (and middle school) sports participation. A thorough evaluation is important before matriculating into a specific sport, whether at the elementary school, middle school, high school, college, or professional level. Annual re-evaluations thereafter often are less comprehensive if there are no changes in an athlete's health status. The initial PPE is usually performed 4 to 6 weeks before a new athletic season begins.

## 4   Cardiac Evaluation

The cardiac evaluation is an essential part of the PPE, but how extensive it should be is controversial.

Cardiovascular risk assessment has been the focus of much attention over the years because of the rare but highly publicized cases of "sudden death" syndromes, in which a seemingly strong and healthy young individual fatally collapses during or immediately after sports participation. The actual incidence of sudden death is very rare, 0.2 to 0.5 deaths per 100,000 adolescents per year. It is usually caused by structural heart defects in athletes under 30 years of age, or coronary artery disease in athletes over 30 years of age.

Cardiac screening of all athletes (including tests such as electrocardiograms, stress tests, and echocardiograms) for sudden death syndromes is thought by many to be cost prohibitive and not cost effective, due to the rather low yield of positive results. The decision whether or not a particular team or league performs extensive cardiac screening exams is widely individualized. The screening process should, however, begin by asking simple questions about personal and family risk factors (Table 1.1). If key risk factors are identified, further diagnostic tests and cardiology consultations are appropriate.

### 4.1   Key Cardiovascular Risk Factors

1. Family history of heart disease.
2. Persistent high blood pressure (upper limits of normal: 130/75 in children less than 10 years old, 140/85 in children over 10).
3. Smoking history.
4. High cholesterol (elevated serum total and LDL cholesterol and low serum HDL cholesterol).
5. Diabetes history.
6. History of cardiac symptoms: palpitations, dizziness/collapse, shortness of breath, or chest pain.

**Table 1.1** Preparticipation physical evaluation

| | | | | | |
|---|---|---|---|---|---|
| Name _____ | Sex _____ | Age _____ | Date of Birth _____ |

Name _____ Sex _____ Age _____ Date of Birth _____
Grade _____ School _____ Sport (s) _____
Address _____ Phone _____
Personal physician _____
In case of emergency, contact
Name _____ Relationship _____ Phone _____

HISTORY

Explain "Yes" answers. Circle questions you don't know answers to.

1. Have you had a medical illness or injury since your last check up or sports physical?
2. Do you have an ongoing or chronic illness?
3. Have you ever been hospitalized overnight?
4. Have you ever had surgery?
5. Are you taking prescription or nonprescription (over-the-counter) meds or pills or using an inhaler?
6. Do you take supplements of vitamins to gain/lose weight or improve performance?
7. Do you have allergies (i.e., pollen, medicine, food, and stinging insects)?
8. Have you ever had rashes or hives develop during or after exercise?
9. Have you ever passed out during exercise?
10. Have you ever been dizzy during or after exercise?
11. Have you ever had chest pain during or after exercise?
12. Do you get tired more quickly than your friends during exercise?
13. Have you ever had racing of your heart or skipped heartbeats?
14. Have you ever had high blood pressure or cholesterol?
15. Have you ever been told you have a heart murmur?
16. Has any family member or relative died of heart problems or of sudden death before age 50?
17. Have you had a severe viral infection (i.e., myocarditis or mononucleosis) within the last month?
18. Has a physician ever denied or restricted your participation in sports for any heart problems?
19. Do you have any current skin problems (i.e., itching, rashes, acne, warts, fungus, or blisters)?
20. Have you ever had a head injury or concussion?
21. Have you ever been knocked out, become unconscious, or lost your memory?
22. Have you ever had a seizure?
23. Do you have frequent or severe headaches? Have you ever had numbness or tingling in your arms, hands, legs, or feet?
24. Have you ever had a stinger, burner, or pinched nerve?
25. Have you ever become ill from exercising in the heat?
26. Do you cough, wheeze, or have trouble breathing during or after activity?
27. Do you have asthma?
28. Do you have seasonal allergies that require medical treatment?
29. Do you use any special protection or corrective equipment or devices that aren't normally used?
30. Have you had any problems with your eyes or vision?
31. Do you wear glasses, contacts, or protective eyewear?
32. Have you ever had a sprain, strain, or swelling after injury?
33. Have you broken or fractured any bones or dislocated any joints?
34. Have you had any other problems with pain or swelling in muscles, tendons, bones, or joints?
35. *If yes, check appropriate box and explain below.*

| | | |
|---|---|---|
| i. Head | Elbow | Hip |
| ii. Neck | Forearm | Thigh |
| iii. Back | Wrist | Knee |

|   |   |   |
|---|---|---|
| iv. Chest | Hand | Shin/calf |
| v. Shoulder | Finger | Ankle |
| vi. Upper arm | Foot | |

36. Do you want to weight more or less than you do now?
37. Do you lose weight regularly to meet weight requirements for your sport?
38. Do you feel stressed out?
39. Record the dates of your most recent immunizations

    i. Tetanus _____    Measles _____
   ii. Hepatitis B _____    Chickenpox _____

## FEMALES ONLY

1. When was you first menstrual period?
2. When was your most recent period?
3. How much time do you usually have from the start of one period to the start of another?
4. How many periods have you had in the last year?
5. What was the longest time between periods in the last year?

## PHYSICAL EXAM

Name _____ Date of birth _____
Height _____ Weight _____ Pulse _____ BP _____
Vision _____ R 20/ _____ L 20/ _____ Corrected: Y/N _____ Pupils: Equal ____ Unequal____
**Appearance: Nl or ABN (Please explain all abnormals below)**

|   |   |   |
|---|---|---|
| Eyes/Ears/Nose/Throat | Neck | Leg/ ankle |
| Lymph Nodes | Back | Foot |
| Pulses | Shoulder/arm | |
| Lungs | Elbow/forearm | |
| Abdomen | Wrist/hand | |
| Genitalia (males only) | Hip/thigh | |
| Skin | Knee | |

_____
_____
_____

## CLEARANCE

- Cleared without restrictions
- Cleared after completing evaluation/ rehabilitation for:
- Not cleared for:         Reason:

Recommendations_____
_____
_____
_____

Name of physician _____
Address _____
Telephone _____ Fax _____
Signature of physician _____ MD/DO _____ Date _____

Sample preparticipation evaluation. Reprinted from American Academy of Family Physicians, American Academy of Pediatrics, American Medical Society for Sports Medicine, American Orthopaedic Society for Sports Medicine, American Osteopathic Academy of Sports Medicine (1997) Preparticipation physical evaluation, 2nd edn. The Physician and Sports Medicine, McGraw-Hill, Minneapolis

## 4.2 Cardiac Contraindications for Sports Participation

1. Hypertrophic cardiomyopathy
2. Congenital coronary artery abnormalities
3. Severe pulmonic stenosis or aortic stenosis
4. Long QT syndromes
5. Active myocarditis or pericarditis
6. Marfan's syndrome

# 5 Pulmonary Evaluation

While evaluating the athlete for any wheezes or evidence of acute pulmonary infection, there are a few pulmonary conditions that require attention. Controlled asthma is not a contraindication for athletic participation. A physician's note, including documentation for the use of a hand-held inhaler is required for athletes with asthma. Most athletes with severe pulmonary compromise are discouraged from participating in high-intensity sports, while the majority are cleared for low-intensity sports participation (see Table 1.1).

## 5.1 Pulmonary Risks Factors for Sports Participation

1. Uncontrolled severe asthma (well-controlled asthma and exercise-induced asthma are not contraindicated)
2. Serious pulmonary infections (i.e., tuberculosis)
3. Conditions that compromise an athlete's respiratory status (i.e., cystic fibrosis or COPD)

# 6 Neurological Evaluation

Like the cardiac evaluation, a thorough history is important (refer to Table 1.2, Question 7). There are well-established guidelines for grading and managing concussions, both on and off the field. It is crucial to understand these guidelines in order to prevent serious brain injury such as "second impact" syndrome. Any loss of consciousness during contact/collision sports warrants immediate attention and neurological imaging. Temporary nerve root injuries or traction injuries to the brachial plexus results (i.e., "stingers" or "burners") usually resolve on their own. Persistent upper extremity numbness or weakness warrants cervical spine imaging.

**Table 1.2** Common sports classifications

A. Classification of sports by contact

| Contact/collision | Limited contact | Noncontact |
|---|---|---|
| Basketball | Baseball | Aerobics |
| Boxing | Bicycling | Archery |
| Diving | Cheerleading | Badminton |
| Field hockey | Canoeing/kayaking | Body building |
| Football | Fencing | Bowling |
| Ice hockey | Field (high jump/pole vault) | Crew/rowing |
| Lacrosse | Gymnastics | Dancing |
| Martial arts | Handball | Golf |
| Rodeo | Horseback riding | Power/weight lifting |
| Rugby | Skating | Running/track |
| Ski jumping | Skiing | Sailing |
| Water polo | Softball | Swimming |
| Wrestling | Ultimate Frisbee | Tennis |
| | Squash/racquetball | |
| | Volleyball | |
| | Surfing | |

B. Classification of sports by strenuousness

| Dynamic & static demands | Static demands | Dynamic demands |
|---|---|---|
| High to moderate intensity | | |
| Boxing | Badminton | Archery |
| Crew/rowing | Baseball | Diving |
| Cross-country skiing | Basketball | Field events |
| Fencing | Lacrosse | Gymnastics |
| Football | Ping-pong | Martial arts |
| Ice hockey | Racquetball | Sailing |
| Rugby | Soccer | Ski jumping |
| Speed skating | Squash | Waterskiing |
| Water polo | Swimming | Weight lifting |
| Wrestling | Tennis | |
| Low intensity | | |
| Bowling | | |
| Cricket | | |
| Golf | | |
| Curling | | |
| Riflery | | |

Adapted from American Academy of Pediatrics Committee on Sports Medicine and Fitness (1994) Medical conditions affecting sports participation. Pediatrics 94:391

## 6.1 Neurological Risk Factors

1. History of concussions
2. Traumatic brain injury
3. Seizures

## 6.2 Contraindications for Further Participation in Contact/Collision Sports

Contraindications for further participation in contact/collision sports include persistent postconcussive symptoms (i.e., headache, dizziness, mental status changes, memory loss, and sensory impairments).

## 6.3 Absolute Contraindications to Participation in Contact Sports

1. History of craniotomy
2. The presence of a large cranial defect
3. Uncontrolled seizure disorders

# 7 Musculoskeletal Evaluation

The PPE is likely to be centered on the musculoskeletal system (Table 1.3). It is important to focus the exam on the body parts most at risk, depending on the sport and the athlete's personal history of injuries. The examiner should begin with an accurate and detailed history of all injuries. Knees, ankles, and shoulders have been shown to be most at risk, depending on the sport. Acute injuries should be evaluated carefully. One good indicator that a player may return to his or her sport is if the player can simulate sports-specific exercises without acute symptoms.

# 8 Athletes with Organ Loss or Impairment

Athletes with one kidney who have undergone organ transplant or have chronic organ enlargement need individual assessment before clearance for contact/collision sports. An athlete with acute organ enlargement (such as an enlarged spleen from EBV mononucleosis) may not be cleared for contact/collision sports.

Athletes with one functional eye must take special precautions to protect the intact eye, and must realize that depth perception is decreased, making them more prone to injury. Athletes who have undergone eye surgery or serious eye injury likewise need special protective eye gear. Sports involving a puck or ball carry an increased risk for these individuals.

**Table 1.3** Two-minute musculoskeletal examination

| Athletic activity (instructions) | Observations |
|---|---|
| 1. Stand facing examiner | Acromioclavicular joints, general habitus |
| 2. Look at ceiling, floor, over both shoulders; touch ears to shoulders | Cervical spine motion |
| 3. Shrug shoulders (examiner resists) | Trapezius strength |
| 4. Abduct shoulders 90 degrees (examiner resists at 90 degrees) | Deltoid strength |
| 5. Full external rotation of arms | Shoulder motion |
| 6. Flex and extend elbows | Elbow motion |
| 7. Arms at sides, elbows at 90 degrees flexed; pronate and supinate wrists | Elbow and wrist motion |
| 8. Spread fingers; make fist | Hand and finger motion and deformities |
| 9. Tighten quadriceps; relax quadriceps | Symmetry and knee effusion, ankle effusion |
| 10. "Duck walk" four steps away | Hip, knee, and ankle motion (Fig. 1.1) |

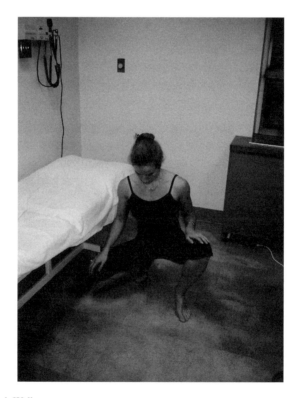

**Fig. 1.1** Duck Walk

| 11. Back to examiner | Shoulder symmetry, scoliosis |
|---|---|
| 12. Knees straight, touch toes | Scoliosis, hip motion, hamstring tightness |
| 13. Raise up on toes, heels | Calf symmetry, leg strength |

Adapted from McKeag D (1989) Preparticipation screening of the potential athlete. Clin Sports Med 8:391

# 9 Other Important Medical Conditions to Consider in Sports Participation

There are a multitude of medical conditions that may require special consideration during the PPE, depending on the individual's needs and the sport involved. For example, diabetic athletes need to pay special attention to hydration, diet, and insulin therapy. Sickle cell disease patients may be allowed limited participation of noncontact/noncollision sports, but must avoid overheating, dehydration, and chilling.

Active infection is another problem. Fever and diarrhea are indications for postponing an athlete's participation in sports due to the risk of heat illness, dehydration, and orthostatic hypotension, all of which make exercise dangerous.

Certain conditions, including HIV and various skin conditions (i.e., herpes simplex, impetigo, scabies, and molluscum contagiosum), may cause concern for other athletes. Athletes with these skin conditions should avoid sports involving mats and cover all skin lesions. Athletic personnel should always use universal precautions when handling blood or body fluids with visible blood.

# 10 How Is Illegal Drug Use Assessed?

Unfortunately, cigarette smoking, alcohol, and other drugs are seen among athletes just as they are among the general population. One should always ask about drugs in the routine health history of a patient. Whether or not a urine specimen is necessary to rule out drugs is case sensitive. At the professional and college level, athletes are required to undergo routine urine testing.

Sometimes there are physical clues of drug abuse—such as unexplained seizures, high blood pressure, and rapid or abnormal pulses—which may be the result of cocaine abuse. Pupil size in another important clue in the acute drug overdose setting. Evidence of anabolic steroid use, "blood doping," or other such practices unfortunately is more difficult to assess on exam alone. Disproportionate muscular hypertrophy or male secondary sex characteristics in the female athlete may provide hints of steroid use.

# 11 Female Athletes

The evaluation of female athletes requires certain considerations. Questions geared toward eating habits and menstrual cycle are important. Also, insuring the use of proper equipment such as chest protectors while boxing should not be disregarded.

It is important to be able to recognize the "female athletic triad," which occurs most often in gymnastics, running, and dancing. This triad of amenorrhea, eating disorders, and anemia may be overlooked, especially for athletes who are guarded about revealing personal habits.

## 12   Disabled Athletes

There are approximately two to three million athletes in the United States with physical and mental disabilities who participate in organized sports. It is important to be sensitive to the ethical and legal issues involved with this population, as well as their particular risk factors. For example, patients with severe lupus and rheumatoid arthritis, who may or may not be on steroid treatment, are prone to injuries from weakened tendons and capsular structures. Athletes with rheumatoid arthritis are also at risk due to possible neck instability and should avoid collision/contact sports, diving, and swimming breast/butterfly strokes.

Athletes with spinal cord injuries have their own set of medical concerns. For example, shoulder injuries and carpal tunnel syndrome are very common among the wheelchair-dependent population. Exercises that strengthen the rotator cuff and scapular stabilizers should be initiated early. Also, paralyzed athletes can accumulate fluid in the immobilized extremities during physical activity, which diminishes cardiac return and cardiac output. These individuals should be advised to use compressive garments during exercise. Paraplegic athletes with high thoracic injuries (above the T6 neurological level) have problems regulating body temperature and should be advised to avoid exposure to severe environments. There are also skin issues of potential concern, such as pressure sores, and persistent fungal infections which must be identified and addressed.

There are a multitude of committees representing the disabled athlete, such as the Committee on Sports for the Disabled, the United States Cerebral Palsy Athletic Association, and the Special Olympics. Patients should be aware of these groups and know how to contact them for more information.

## References

1. Alliance for the Advancement of Clinical Sports Medicine (2001) Sideline preparedness for the team physician: a consensus statement. Med Sci Sports Exerc 33(5):846–849
2. American Academy of Pediatrics' Committee on Sports Medicine and Fitness (1994) Medical conditions affecting sports participation. Pediatrics 94:391
3. American Academy of Family Physicians, American Academy of Pediatrics, American Medical Society for Sports Medicine, American Orthopaedic Society for Sports Medicine, American Osteopathic Academy of Sports Medicine. (1997) The physician and sports medicine, 2nd ed. McGraw-Hill, New York
4. Best TM (2004) The preparticipation evaluation: an opportunity for change and consensus. Cl J Sports Med 14(3):107–108
5. Braddom RL (2000) Physical medicine and rehabilitation. In: Laskowski ER, Braddom ER, Randall L (eds.) Concepts in sports medicine, 2nd ed. WB Saunders, Philadelphia
6. International Olympics Committee, USA (1993) Sports injuries: basic principles of prevalence and care
7. Kurowski K (2000) The preparticipation evaluation. American Academy of Family Physicians. Am Fam Phys 61:2683–2690, 2696–2698
8. Magnes SA et al. (1992) What conditions limit sports participation? Phys Sports Med 20(5):143–160

9. Maron BJ, Thompson PD, Puffer JC et al. (1996) Cardiovascular preparticipation screening of competitive athletes: a statement for health professionals from the Sudden Death Committee and Congenital Cardiac Defects Committee. Am Heart Assoc 94:850–856

10. McGrew CA (1999) Handbook of sports medicine, 2nd edn. Butterworth-Heinemann, Burlington, MA

11. McKeag D (1989) Preparticipation screening of the potential athlete. Clin Sports Med 8:391

12. Mick TM, Dimeff RJ (2004) What kind of physical exam does a young athlete need before participation in sports? Cleveland Clin J Med 71:7

13. Miller MJ (1996) When is disqualification from sports justified? Medical judgment vs. patient's rights. Phys Sports Med 24:10

14. Mitchell JH et al. (1985) Cardiovascular abnormalities in the athlete: recommendations regarding eligibility for competition. J Am Coll Cardiol 6:1186–1232

15. Paterick T, Fletcher G, Maron B et al. (2005) Medical and legal issues in cardiovascular evaluation of competitive athletes. JAMA 294:3011–3018

16. Press J, Young J (1997) PM&R secrets: sports medicine. Hanley and Belfus, Philadelphia

17. Sallis R (1997) ACSM's essentials of sports medicine. American College of Sports Medicine, Indianapolis

18. Smith D, Morris BM (eds.) (1996) The preparticipation evaluation of young athletes. Hanley and Belfus, Philadelphia

19. Tanner JM (1962) Growth at adolescence; with a general consideration of the effects of hereditary and environmental factors upon growth and maturation from birth to maturity, 2nd edn. Blackwell Scientific, Oxford

20. Taylor W, Lombardo J (1990) Preparticipation screening of college athletes: value of the CBC. Phys Sports Med 18(6)106–118

21. U.S. Preventive Service Task Force (1996) Guide to clinical preventive services, 2nd ed. Williams & Wilkins, Baltimore

22. Van Camp SP et al. (1995) Nontraumatic sports death in high school and college athletes. Med Sci Sports Exerc 27:641–647

23. Wingfield K et al. (2004) Preparticipation physician evaluation: An evidence-based Review. Cl J Sports Med 14(3):109–122 available at www.clevelandclinic.org/health/health.info/docs/0400/451.asp

# Chapter 2
# Traumatic Brain Injury in Sports

**Danielle Marie Perret and Barry D. Jordan**

## 1  Introduction

Few physicians realize the detriment and prevalence of head injury in the athlete. Due to the development of organized athletics with more standardized rules, which help to decide how head injury should be managed and when players should return to play, and due to the development of newer and better protective equipment, fatal and near-fatal head injuries have been declining. Still, mild traumatic brain injury or concussion is under-recognized and continues to have a significant impact on the future well-being of the athlete. Given the tremendous popularity of sports in the United States and the world, there are large numbers of athletes—competitive and recreational—who sustain mild traumatic brain injury. In 1997, The Centers for Disease Control and Prevention had already proclaimed that concussions had reached epidemic proportions in the United States. Further, there is accumulating evidence that mild traumatic brain injury, including sports-related concussion, may be more common and more devastating than previously considered.

Traumatic brain injury (TBI) in sports is relatively uncommon occurrence that may be associated with significant morbidity and occasional mortality. Although TBI in sports is infrequent, certain contact/collision and high velocity sports have an increased risk of TBI (Table 2.1). There are several brain injury syndromes that can be encountered in sports. These include acute traumatic brain injury (ATBI), the second impact syndrome (SIS) and chronic traumatic brain injury (CTBI). ATBI represents the immediate effects of traumatic forces involving the brain, whereas CTBI represents the more long-term cumulative effects of traumatic forces to the brain. The SIS is a syndrome in which an athlete who sustains a second TBI while still symptomatic from an initial concussion and experiences malignant cerebral edema and herniation. These three categories of TBI are discussed in detail.

J.E. Herrera and G. Cooper (eds.), *Essential Sports Medicine,*
doi: 10.1007/978-1-59745-414-8, © Humana Press 2008

**Table 2.1** Sports associated with increased risk of traumatic brain injury

Contact/collision sports
Boxing
Football
Field hockey
Ice hockey
Lacrosse
Martial arts
Rugby and Australian rules football
Soccer
Wrestling

High-velocity sports
Auto racing
Cycling
Equestrian sports
Roller skating/roller blading
Rodeo
Skateboarding
Skiing/snowboarding

# 2    Acute Traumatic Brain Injury

Pathologically, ATBI can be classified into four major categories: skull fractures, diffuse brain injury, focal brain injury, and penetrating brain injury (Table 2.2). Skull fractures are relatively infrequent in sports unless associated with the unprotected head striking a hard surface (e.g., railing, goalpost, tree, ground, playing surface) especially in high-velocity sports (e.g., skiing, cycling). The presence of a skull fracture often implies a high-energy impact. Diffuse injuries include cerebral concussion and diffuse axonal injury (DAI). Concussion is defined as a complex pathophysiological process affecting the brain, induced by traumatic biomechanical forces. Other characteristics of concussion are listed in Table 2.3. In geneal a concussion is considered to be a functional rather than structural dysfunction of the brain assiciated with negative neuroimaging. DAI is characterized by post-traumatic coma lasting 6 hours or longer in the absence of focal lesions on brain imaging. Patients experiencing DAI may remain in coma from days to weeks. Shearing injury to the white matter tracts more typically occur in the midbrain-diencephalon, cerebral hemispheres, corpus callosum, and the cerebellar peduncles causing punctate hemorrhages and edema. Focal injuries include epidural hematoma, subdural hematoma, cerebral contusion, intracerebral hemorrhage, subarachnoid hemorrhage, and intraventricular hemorrhage. DAI and focal brain injuries usually present as moderate to severe brain injuries and are also relatively uncommon in sports. Penetrating injuries are those injuries in which foreign objects or missiles penetrate the calvarium and brain. In sports these types of injuries are relatively uncommon.

**Table 2.2** Pathological classification of acute traumatic brain injury in sports

A. Diffuse brain injury
    1. Cerebral concussion
    2. Diffuse axonal injury
B. Focal brain injury
    1. Epidural hematoma
    2. Subdural hematoma
    3. Cerebral contusion
    4. Intracerebral hemorrhage
    5. Subarachnoid hemorrhage
    6. Intraventricular hemorrhage
C. Skull fracture
D. Penetrating brain injury

**Table 2.3** Characteristics of concussion

1. May be caused by a direct blow to the head, face, neck, or elsewhere on the body with an "impulsive" force transmitted to the head
2. Typically results in the rapid onset short-lived impairment of neurological function that resolves spontaneously
3. May result in pathological changes but acute clinical symptoms largely reflect a functional disturbance rather than a structural injury
4. Results in a graded set of clinical syndromes that may or may not involve loss of consciousness. Resolution of the clinical and cognitive symptoms typically follows a sequential course
5. Typically associated with grossly normal structural neuroimaging studies

## 2.1 Clinical Presentation

Clinically, ATBI can be further classified according to clinical severity as mild, moderate, or severe according to the Glasgow Coma Scale (Tables 2.4 and 2.5). Generally speaking MTBI (GCS score 13–15) is synonymous with the cerebral concussion and these terms are often used interchangeably in the clinical literature. However, on occasion an individual may present clinically as a concussion but may exhibit focal brain pathology (e.g., contusion, subdural hematoma) on neuroimaging. These types of cases are often classified as complicated MTBI, but the more accurate classification should be based on the pathological description. Moderate/severe TBI (GCS score 3–12) are infrequent in sports and are more often associated with focal brain injury and/or DAI. Although the GCS is relatively insensitive in assessing concussion or MTBI, it provides a general framework for acute management and triage of a brain traumatized athlete.

An athlete that experiences a concussion or MTBI may present with a variety of cognitive, behavioral, and physical signs and symptoms (Table 2.6). Common symptoms include headache, amnesia, and confusion. Concussion can occur in the absence of LOC (loss of consciousness). When a LOC does occur, it tends to be of short duration (less than a minute). Athletes with a prolonged duration of LOC several minutes or more may be harboring a more severe brain injury that may

**Table 2.4** Glasgow Coma Scale

| Response | | Score |
|---|---|---|
| Verbal | None | 1 |
| | Incomprehensible sounds | 2 |
| | Inappropriate words | 3 |
| | Confused | 4 |
| | Oriented | 5 |
| Eye opening | None | 1 |
| | To pain | 2 |
| | To speech | 3 |
| | Spontaneously | 4 |
| Motor | None | 1 |
| | Abnormal extension | 2 |
| | Abnormal flexion | 3 |
| | Withdraws | 4 |
| | Localizes | 5 |
| | Obeys | 6 |

**Table 2.5** Clinical classification of traumatic brain injury

| |
|---|
| Mild: GCS* score 13–15 |
| Moderate: GCS score 9–12 |
| Severe: GCS score 3–8 |

*GCS Glasgow Coma Scale

necessitate more emergent treatment. The postconcussion syndrome represents persistent symptoms following a concussion and may include: persistent headache, irritability, inability to concentrate, dizziness, vertigo, memory impairment, generalized fatigue, changes in mood, cognitive deficits, depression, and anxiety. Postconcussion syndrome in the athlete is usually self-limited, lasting approximately 7–10 days. However, athletes may underreport or minimize any neurological or cognitive symptoms in order to return to competition.

Athletes that present with a moderate to severe brain injury (i.e., GCS score 3–12) will present with more ominous neurological signs and symptoms that require more immediate neurological attention (Table 2.7). In particular, athletes with prolonged LOC especially with delayed recovery of alertness and decreased level of arousal should be suspected of experiencing a more severe brain injury. Other serious signs and symptoms include focal weakness, seizures (not impact seizures), and cranial nerve palsies.

## 2.2 Pathophysiology

ATBI may result from direct impact or impulse insults to the head. Impact injuries occur when a mass strikes the head and transmits kinetic energy to the skull and brain, whereas impulse injuries occur when there is no direct impact to the head but

**Table 2.6** Common signs and symptoms of acute concussion

Cognitive features
Decreased speed of information processing
Disorientation
Unawareness
Confusion
Amnesia/memory impairment
Impaired concentration
Loss of consciousness

Behavioral features
Sleep disturbance
Irritability
Emotional lability
Nervousness/anxiety
Psychomotor retardation
Apathy
Fatigue
Easy distractibility

Physical features
Headache
Dizziness/vertigo
Nausea
Vacant stare
Impaired playing ability
Gait unsteadiness/loss of balance
Impaired coordination
Diplopia
Photophobia
Hyperacusis
Concussive convulsion/impact seizure

**Table 2.7** Indications for neurological evaluation following a traumatic brain injury in sports

Glasgow Coma Scale score of 3–12
Loss of consciousness associated with delayed recovery of function
Persistent neurological symptoms lasting longer than 24 hours
Focal neurological deficits (e.g., hemiparesis, hemisensory loss, aphasia, or unilateral
    hyperreflexia)
Seizures (focal or generalized), not including impact seizures
Clinical evidence of skull fracture (e.g., Battle's sign, raccoon eyes, or cranial nerve palsies)

instead there are abrupt changes in head movement resulting in acceleration and deceleration of the brain. Impact injuries typically produce focal injuries. The primary mechanism of traumatic brain injury in sports is the rapid acceleration and deceleration of the head by mechanical forces. There are three types of acceleration including rotational (angular), linear (translational), and impact deceleration. Among these, rotational acceleration is considered the primary culprit in producing brain injury. The sports that rank highest in brain injury (e.g., football, boxing, and

**Table 2.8** Molecular mechanisms in the pathophysiology of traumatic brain injury

| |
| --- |
| Glutamate toxicity |
| Ionic alterations |
| Inflammatory responses |
| Cholinergic dysfunction |
| Growth factor alterations |
| Apoptosis |
| Calpain/caspase activation |
| Mitochondrial dysfunction |
| Free radical formation and peroxidation |

ice hockey) all involve a high amount of acceleration-deceleration forces in the form of punches, blocks, and tackles. Rotatory energy forces cause impulsive rather than impact loading forces and these are thought to cause more shearing and tensile stresses to the cerebral tissue. Trauma to the brain initiates a pathophysiological cascade of molecular and neurometabolic events (Table 2.8). These include neurotransmitter changes, ionic alterations, metabolic dysfunction, apoptosis, and inflammatory processes. A full discussion of these events is beyond the scope of this chapter; however, the reader is referred to the text of Miller and Hayes for a comprehensive review.

## 2.3 Diagnosis and Management

Any athlete who sustains direct or indirect trauma to the head and exhibits new cognitive and/or neurological symptoms should be considered to have sustained a traumatic brain insult until proven otherwise. In the unconscious athlete the initial examination must involve the basic principles of cardiopulmonary resuscitation. If a player is unconscious, the player should be assumed to have a spinal cord or vertebral column injury. Therefore, the airway should be properly maintained and safe transport off the field must be determined. Although in athletes, unconsciousness is usually brief, lasting only seconds to minutes, any prolonged unconsciousness similarly requires transport off the field to the nearest trauma center for full neurosurgical evaluation.

The neurological examination should begin with an assessment for the level of consciousness. The neurological examination should then continue with a cranial nerve exam and a motor, sensory and reflexes examination; a detailed examination should be repeated once the patient has been transported off the field. The examination of the athlete with a concussion should also include a detailed mental status examination. This should include: orientation to person, place, and time; assessment of immediate, recent, and remote memory; assessment of the ability to solve simple calculations; and assessment of abstract reasoning. The mental status examination can be performed within as little as 2–3 minutes and is invaluable. It can be easily reproduced to provide a dynamic picture of the head injury, assisting in the decision for further medical diagnosis and care and assisting in the decision of the physician or coach for return to play of the athlete.

Any athlete who sustains a moderate or severe brain injury (i.e., GCS 3–12) should be transported to the emergency room for further evaluation and treatment. Signs and symptoms of more serious neurological injury are listed in Table 2.7. Individuals that experience a moderate or severe TBI will typically exhibit focal findings on neurological examination and will have an altered level of consciousness. Any athlete with a GCS score of 8 or less will be in a coma.

Neuroimaging provides a useful adjunct in the evaluation of the athlete with ATBI. Although in concussion or MTBI computed tomographic (CT) scanning and magnetic resonance imaging (MRI) may be negative, these tests are useful in ruling out structural brain injuries and provide guidance in the management of moderate and severe brain injuries. In general the MRI scan is more sensitive than CT in detecting white matter lesions, cerebral contusions, or small subdural hematomas.

Neuropsychological testing may provide useful information in the assessment of the athlete with ATBI. Neuropsychological testing also allows the medical community to follow the evolution of cognitive and higher cortical deficits after a brain injury. A baseline preseason neuropsychological exam is recommended and includes tests on orientation, attention, memory, and information processing, among others. These tests may be repeated as early as 48 hours after a head injury. Usually, an uncomplicated concussion will have findings that revert to normal within 7 to 10 days. However, even mild abnormalities on exam indicate that there is an ongoing or persistent effect of the brain injury. An additive association between multiple episodes of concussion and learning disabilities has been demonstrated.

## 2.4   Return to Competition

According to the Summary Statement of the Second International Conference on Concussion in Sport, whether an athlete returns to competition should be determined on an individual basis. Although there have been several published guidelines for return to competition following concussion there has been a more recent trend to abandon these guidelines. Return to competition should follow a stepwise progression (Table 2.9). No athlete should return to competition while still symptomatic from a concussion or MTBI. Currently there are no established guidelines for return to competition following moderate to severe TBI or complicated MTBI. Obviously any athlete who exhibits persistent neurological symptoms or evidence of traumatic neuropathology (e.g., residual hemorrhage) should not return to contact collision sports.

**Table 2.9** Stepwise approach to return to play following concussion

1. No activity, complete rest. Once asymptomatic, proceed to next step
2. Light aerobic exercise such as walking or stationary cycling, no resistance training
3. Sport specific exercise with progressive addition of resistance training
4. Noncontact training drills with progressive addition of resistance training
5. Full contact training after medical clearance
6. Game play

# 3   Second Impact Syndrome

Second-impact syndrome is a rare but potentially fatal cumulative injury that occurs when an athlete, having not yet recovered from an acute brain injury, sustains a second injury before the symptoms associated with the first injury have resolved. This syndrome dramatizes the extreme vulnerability of the mildly injured brain. The true incidence of SIS is actually unknown. The National Center for Catastrophic Sports Injury Research reported 35 probable cases during the time period of 1980 through 1993 and 17 of these were confirmed with necropsy or surgery and MRI findings. The SIS has been reported in football, boxing, ice hockey, and downhill skiing.

## 3.1   Clinical Presentation

Before the symptoms of one concussion resolve, the athlete returns to play and then sustains another head injury, which in fact may even be a mild blow to the head or even a blow to the chest, that indirectly jerks and accelerates the head. Within a few seconds to minutes of this second impact, the athlete, who is still conscious, collapses to the ground and becomes comatose. Rapidly dilating pupils, loss of eye movement and respiratory failure usually ensue. SIS has a mortality rate near 50% and a morbidity rate near 100%. For this reason, knowledge and respect of the proper management of head injury in the athlete is crucial. Any player who sustains a head injury must not be allowed to return to play until all of his or her symptoms have fully resolved.

## 3.2   Pathophysiology

The SIS is believed to result from loss of the brain's auto regulatory function. Vascular engorgement and intracranial hypertension follow with the ultimate result of uncal or cerebellar herniation, or both. This may lead to respiratory failure and often death.

## 3.3 Diagnosis and Management

The majority of times SIS will present as a moderate or severe TBI in the setting of a rather trivial head trauma in an athlete who is experiencing a postconcussion syndrome. The management of an athlete experiencing the SIS would first require cardiopulmonary resuscitation followed by emergent neurological evaluation (see management of moderate and severe TBI above).

## 3.4 Return to Competition

Return to competition following the SIS is not advisable secondary to high mortality rate and severe morbidity associated with the condition. Currently there are no established guidelines for return to competition following the SIS. If an athlete does survive the SIS, then multidisciplinary rehabilitation and reintegration into society following this catastrophic neurological event will be the primary concern.

# 4 Chronic Traumatic Brain Injury

CTBI has been a disorder more commonly reported among boxers; however, this condition can also be encountered in football, ice hockey, soccer, rugby, and potentially any sport associated with recurrent concussion. The frequency of CTBI in sports is largely unknown. It has been estimated that the prevalence of CTBI among retired professional boxers is 17%; however, the incidence or prevalence in football, ice hockey, soccer, rugby and other contact collision sports is unknown. Cumulative injury is an extremely important concept in athletic concussion. There can be significant morbidity associated with more than one concussive episode. After a second concussion, the postconcussion syndrome is more pronounced. Multiple concussions may affect personality, academic performance, and the ability to return to competition. However, long-term effects can be even more devastating.

## 4.1 Clinical Presentation

CTBI has been best studied in boxers and first described as early as 1928 to include advanced parkinsonism, pyramidal tract dysfunction, ataxia, and behavioral abnormalities. End stages may also include severe cerebellar, cognitive, and psychiatric abnormalities, often termed *dementia pugilistica,* and are associated with several characteristic pathology findings in brains. The presence of the apolipoprotein E €4 allele seems to be associated with more severe CTBI.

Signs and symptoms of CTBI associated with boxing can involve motor, cognitive and/or behavioral impairments (Table 2.10). Early motor impairments may

**Table 2.10** Common signs and symptoms of chronic traumatic brain injury

| |
|---|
| Cognitive |
| Decreased attention |
| Executive dysfunction |
| Memory impairment |
| Dementia |
| Behavioral |
| Emotional lability |
| Euphoria/hypomania |
| Inappropriate violent outbursts |
| Disinhibition/poor impulse control |
| Psychosis |
| Impaired insight/poor judgment |
| Motor |
| Dysarthria, scanning speech |
| Incoordination, ataxia |
| Spasticity |
| Parkinsonism |

include mild dysarthria and mild difficulty with balance. As the motor abnormalities progress, the boxer can experience ataxia, spasticity, impaired coordination, and parkinsonism. The parkinsonism encountered in CTBI may be a distinct entity from idiopathic Parkinson's disease. Cognitive impairment in CTBI is most likely to affect attention, memory, and executive/frontal function. Early manifestations of CTBI can include decreased complex attention followed by slowed mental speed and mild deficits in memory, attention, and executive ability. As the disease process advances, the boxer may exhibit dementia exemplified by amnesia, profound attention defects, prominent slowness of thought, and impaired judgment, reasoning, and planning. Behavioral manifestations are an integral component of CTBI and may be difficult to dissociate from premorbid personality characteristics. Behavioral changes encountered can include disinhibition, irritability, euphoria/hypomania, impaired insight, paranoia, and violent outbursts. Debate exists as to whether the behavioral abnormalities occur as an early or late manifestation of the CTBI syndrome. The clinical presentation of CTBI or the effects of cumulative concussion in other sports tends to be less severe than that encountered among boxers and generally is associated with less motor deficits.

## 4.2 Pathophysiology

Although CTBI probably shares several of the pathophysiological mechanisms with ATBI, the pathophysiology has not been elucidated. It has been postulated that cumulative trauma initiates a pathophysiological process that resembles Alzheimer's disease (AD). Similarities between CTBI and AD include amyloid deposition neurofibrillary tangle formation and reduced cholinergic function in the basal forebrain.

## *4.3   Diagnosis and Management*

The diagnosis of CTBI requires a clear documentation of neurological deterioration over time and/or the persistence of neurological symptoms time in the setting of multiple concussions or brain injuries. In severe cases of CTBI (i.e., dementia pugilistica) the athlete will exhibit obvious motor impairment (e.g., dysarthria, incoordination) in addition to cognitive and behavioral manifestations. In milder cases of CTBI only subtle changes in cognitive function may be evident. Accordingly, neuropsychological testing may be instrumental in detecting the cumulative effects of concussion, especially when a preparticipation baseline has been established. In CTBI neuroimaging typically reveals nonspecific findings. CT and MRI scanning may demonstrate brain atrophy with or without a cavum septum pellucidum. Single photon emission computed tomography (SPECT) may exhibit perfusion deficits in boxer that localize primarily to the frontal and temporal regions.

## *4.4   Return to Competition*

The determination whether an athlete should return to competition or terminate participation in a contact/collision sport after experiencing the effects of cumulative concussions can be problematic. Obviously, any athlete that is experiencing persistent cognitive, behavioral, or neurological symptoms as a consequence of repetitive concussions should not be allowed to return to competition. Currently, there are no well-established guidelines when an athlete should terminate a career. Certainly, an athlete who experiences more frequent concussions associated less forceful trauma and experiences longer periods of postconcussion symptoms may consider a modification in activities. There is no established number of concussions that determine when an athlete should terminate a career.

## 5   Discussion

TBI can have devastating effects on the athlete. Accordingly prevention of TBI in sports becomes paramount. Several factors are important in the prevention of TBI in sports (Table 2.11). Education is probably one of the most important factors in the prevention of TBI. First, athletes, trainers, parents, and physicians need to be educated on how to recognize a concussion. It must be recognized that cognitive impairment following head trauma probably represents a concussion at minimum, and the athlete may not experience LOC. The proper recognition of a concussion can prevent more catastrophic injury such as the SIS. The use of helmets, both to spread the force of impact over a larger area and to dissipate kinetic energy via an inner energy absorbing lining, has been the most beneficial in limiting head injury in the athlete,

**Table 2.11** The Prevention of Traumatic Brain Injury in Sports

| |
|---|
| Education |
| Helmet and protective headgear |
| Medical surveillance and preparticipation screening |
| Proper supervision |
| Enforcement of rules and regulations |

especially in high-velocity sports. Another important factor in the prevention of TBI in sports is proper medical surveillance and preparticipation screening. Athletes should undergo a preparticipation medical evaluation to rule out any pre-existing conditions that may predispose that individual to a catastrophic brain injury. The proper medical surveillance should also identify those athletes experiencing a TBI and provide the necessary medical management. Proper conditioning and strengthening, along with full attention to rules and regulations, and their enforcement by trained officials, are also important in preventing head injury.

# References

1. Aubry M, Cantu R, Dvorak J, et al. (2002) Summary and agreement statement of the first international conference on concussion in sport, Vienna 2001. Br J Sports Med 36:6–10, 2002
2. Bailes JE, Cantu RC (2001) Head injury in athletes. Neurosurgery 48:26–46
3. Bailes JE, Hadley MN, Quigley MR, Sonntag VK, Cerullo LJ (1991) Management of athletic injuries of the cervical spine and spinal cord. Neurosurgery 29:491–497
4. Bailes JE, Maroon JC (1996) Neurosurgical trauma in the athlete. In: Tindall GT, Cooper PR, Barrow DL (eds) The practice of neurosurgery. Williams & Wilkins, Baltimore, 1996, pp 1649–1672
5. Barth J, Alves W, Ryan T, Macciocchi S, Rimel R, Jane J, Nelson W (1989) Mild head injury in sports: neuropsychological sequelae and recovery of function. In: Levin H, Eisenberg H, Benton A (eds) Mild head injury. Oxford Press, New York, pp 257–275
6. Barth JT, Macciocchi SN, Giordani B, Rimel R, Jane J, Boll T (1983) Neuropsychological sequelae of minor head injury. Neurosurgery 13:529–533
7. Cantu RC (1986) Guidelines for return to contact sports after a cerebral concussion. Phys Sports Med 14:75–83
8. Cantu RC (1992) Cerebral contusion in sports: management and prevention. Sports Med 14:64–74
9. Cantu RC (1995) Second impact syndrome: a risk in any contact sport. Phys Sports Med 23:27–31
10. Cantu RC (2001) Posttraumatic retrograde and anterograde amnesia: pathophysiology and implications in grading and safe return to play. J Athletic Training 36:244–248
11. Cantu RC, Mueller FO (1999) Fatalities and catastrophic injuries in high school and college sports, 1982–1997. Phys Sports Med 27:35–48
12. Casson IR, Sham R, Campbell EA, et al. (1982) Neurological and CT evaluation of knocked-out boxers. J Neurol Neurosurg Psychiatry 45:170–174
13. Casson IR, Siegel O, Sham R, et al. (1984) Brain damage in modern boxers. JAMA 251:2663–2667
14. Centers for Disease Control and Prevention. (1997) Sports-related recurrent brain injuries, United States. MMWR Morb Mortal Wkly Rep 46:224–227

15. Clarke KS (1998) Epidemiology of athletic head injury. Clin Sports Med 17:1–11
16. Collins MW, Grindel SH, Lovell MR, Dede DE, Moser DJ, Phalin BR, Nogle S, Wasik M, Cordry D, Daugherty MK, Sears SF, Nicolette G, Indelicato P, McKeag DB (1999) Relationship between concussion and neuropsychological performance in college football players. JAMA 282:964–970
17. Corsellis JAN, Bruton CJ, Freeman-Browne C (1973) The aftermath of boxing. Psychol Med 3:270–303
18. Davie CA, Pirtosek Z, Barker GJ, et al. (1995) Magnetic resonance spectroscopic study of parkinsonism related to boxing. J Neurol Neurosurg Psychiatry 58:688–691
19. Gerberich SG, Priest JD, Boen JR, Straub CP, Maxwell RE (1983) Concussion incidences and severity in secondary school varsity football players. Am J Public Health 73:1370–1375
20. Gronwall D, Wrightson P (1983) Cumulative effects of concussion. Lancet 2:995–997, 1975
21. Harris JB (1983) Neurological injuries in winter sports. Phys Sports Med 11:110–122
22. Hugenholtz H, Richard MT (1982) Return to athletic competition following concussion. Can Med Assoc J 127:827–829
23. Jordan BD, Dane SD, Rowen AJ, et al. (1999) SPECT scanning in professional boxers. J Neuroimaging 59–60
24. Jordan SE, Green GA, Galaty H, Mendelbaum BR, Jabour AJ (1996) Acute and chronic brain injury in United States national team soccer players. Acta Neurol Scand 80:151–156
25. Jordan BD, Jahre C, Hauser WA. (1992) Serial computed tomography in professional boxers. Neuroimaging 2:181–185
26. Jordan BD, Jahre C, Hauser WA et al. (1992) CT of 338 active professional boxers. Radiology 185:509–512
27. Jordan BD, Relkin NR, Ravdin LD, Jacobs AR, Bennett A, Gandy S (1997) Apolipoprotein E €4 associated with chronic traumatic brain injury in boxing. JAMA 278:136–140
28. Jordan BD, Tsairis P, Warren RF (eds) (1998) Sports neurology. Lippincott Williams & Wilkins, Philadelphia
29. Jordan BD, Zimmerman RD (1990) Computed tomography, magnetic resonance imaging comparisons in boxers. JAMA 263:1670–1674
30. Junger EC, Newell DW, Grant GA, Avellino AM, Ghatan S, Douville CM, Lam AM, Aaslid R, Winn HR (1997) Cerebral autoregulation following minor head injury. J Neurosurg 86:425–432
31. Kelly JP, Nichols JS, Filley CM, Lillenhei KO, Rubinstein D, Kleinschmidt-DeMasters BK (1991) Concussion in sports: guidelines for the prevention of catastrophic outcome. JAMA 266:2867–2869
32. Kelly JP, Rosenberg JH (1997) Diagnosis and management of concussion in sports. Neurology 48:575–580
33. Kelly JP, Rosenberg JH (1998) The development of guidelines for the management of concussion in sports. J Head Trauma Rehabil 13:53–65
34. Kemp PM, Houston AS, Macleod MA, et al. (1995) Cerebral perfusion and psychometric testing in military amateur boxers and controls. J Neurol Neurosurg Psychol 59:368–374
35. Lampert PW, Hardman JM (1984) Morphological changes in brains of boxers. JAMA 251:2676–2679
36. Lovell MR, Collins MW (1998) Neuropsychological assessment of the college football player. J Head Trauma Rehabil 13:9–26
37. Lovell MR, Maroon JC, Bailes JE, Norwig J (1999) Neuropsychological assessment following minor head injury in professional athletes. In: Bailes JE, Lovell MR, Maroon JC (eds) Sports-related concussion. Quality Medical Publishing, St. Louis, pp 200–228
38. Macciocchi SN, Barth JT, Alves W, Rimel RW, Jane JA (1996) Neuropsychological functioning and recovery after mild head injury in college athletes. Neurosurgery 39:510–514
39. Maddocks DL, Dicker GD, Saling MM (1995) The assessment of orientation following concussion in athletes. Clin J Sport Med 5:32–35
40. Maron BJ, Shirani J, Poliac LC, Mathenge R, Roberts WC, Mueller FO (1996) Sudden death in young competitive athletes: clinical, demographic, and pathological profiles. JAMA 276:199–204

41. Martland HS (1928) Punch drunk. JAMA 91:1103–1107
42. Matser JT, Kessels AG, Lezak MD, Jordan BD, Troost J (1999) Neuro-psychological impairment in amateur soccer players. JAMA 282:971–973
43. McCory P, Johnston K, Meeuwisse W et al. (2005) Summary and agreement statement of the 2nd international conference on concussion in sport, Prague 2004. Clin J Sport Med 15:48–55
44. McCrea M, Kelly JP, Kluge J, Ackley B, Randolph C (1997) Standardized assessment of concussion in football players. Neurology 48:536–538
45. Mendez MF (1995) The neuropsychiatric aspects of boxing. Int J Psychiatry 25:249–262
46. Miller LP, Hayes RL (2001) Head trauma: basic, preclinical, and clinical directions. Wiley-Liss, New York
47. Powell JW, Barber-Foss KD (1999) Traumatic brain injury in high school athletes. JAMA 282:958–963
48. Powell EC, Tang RR (1996) In-line skate and roller skate injuries in childhood. Pediatr Emerg Care 12:259–262
49. Quality Standards Subcommittee, American Academy of Neurology (1997) Practice parameter: the management of concussion in sports (summary statement). Neurology 48:581–585
50. Rabadi MH, Jordan BD (2001) The cumulative effect of repetitive concussion in sports. Clin Journal Sports Med 11:194–198
51. Roberts GW, Allsop D, Bruton C (1990) The occult aftermath of boxing. J Neurol Neurosurg Psychiatr 53:373–378
52. Ross RJ, Cole M Thompson JS, et al. (1983) Boxers—computed tomography, EEG and neurosurgical evaluation. JAMA 249:211–213
53. Saunders RL, Harbaugh RE (1984) The second impact in catastrophic contact sports head trauma. JAMA 252:538–539
54. Schneider RC (1966) Serious and fatal neurosurgical football injuries. Clin Neurosurg 12:226–236
55. Schneider RC, Gosch HH, Norrell H, Jerva M, Combs LW, Smith RA (1970) Vascular insufficiency and differential distortion of brain and cord caused by cervicomedullary football injuries. J Neurosurg 33:363–375
56. Schneider RC, Reifel E, Crisler HO, Oosterbann BG (1961) Serious and fatal football injuries involving the head and spinal cord. JAMA 177:106–111
57. Schneider K, Zernicke RF (1988) Computer simulation of head impact: estimation of head-injury risk during soccer heading. Int J Sport Biomech 4:358–371
58. Sironi VA, Scotti G, Ravagnati L, et al. (1982) CT scan and EEG findings in professional pugilists: early detection of cerebral atrophy in young boxers. J Neurosurg Sci 26:165–168
59. Teasedale G, Jennett B (1974) Assessment of coma and impaired consciousness: a practical scale. Lancet 1:81–84
60. Tokuda T, Ikeda S, Yanugesa N, et al. (1991) Re-examination of ex-boxer's brain using immunohistochemistry with antibodies to amyloid beta protein and tau protein. Acta Neuropathol 82:280–285
61. Uhl GR, McKinney M, Hedreen JC, et al. (1982) Dementia pugilistica: loss of basal forebrain cholinergic neurons and cortical cholinergic markers. Ann Neurol 12:99
62. Warren WL, Bailes JE (1998) On the field evaluation of the athletic head injuries. Clin Sports Med 17:13–26
63. Webbe FM (2006) Definition, physiology, and severity of cerebral concussion. In: Echemendia RJ (ed) Sports neuropsychology. Guilford Press, New York, pp. 45–70
64. Wojtys EM, Hovda D, Landry G, Boland A, Lovell M, McCrea M, Minkoff J (1999) Concussion in sports. Am J Sports Med 27:676–686

# Chapter 3
# Facial Trauma

Fani Thomson and Stephen Gelfman

## 1 Introduction

Maxillofacial injuries occur for a variety of reasons related to sports participation. While most sports-related facial injuries are minor, the potential for serious damage exists. Whether it involves contact between players (head, fist, elbow), with equipment (balls, pucks, handlebars), or with environment, obstacles, or playing surface (wrestling mat, gymnastic equipment, goalposts, trees), fractures of the facial bones require a significant amount of force. A physician examining these injuries must rapidly assess the patient, allowing for prompt diagnosis and appropriate treatment, while considering the physical demands of the sport and the possibility of "return to play."

## 2 Soft Tissue Injuries

In a recent 1-year review of maxillofacial sports injuries, soft tissue injuries were found to be the most common injury. Up to 76% of the athletes reported lacerations. These injuries frequently occur because of poorly designed protective equipment or no protective equipment at all.

Contusions with varying amounts of ecchymosis are the most commonly encountered facial injury. They are due to blunt trauma with subsequent subcutaneous bleeding. In contusions, the overlying skin and mucosa are intact. Ice should be applied immediately to minimize the inflammatory response. Nonsteroidal anti-inflammatory drugs (NSAIDs) can be useful for pain management and swelling but should be used cautiously if significant bleeding may ensue. If the contusion is accompanied by a laceration and wound edge necrosis is expected, the margins may need refinement before closure. Athletes can return to play if their ability to compete safely is not compromised.

Abrasions are superficial disruptions of the epidermis that more commonly overlie prominent facial structures. Deeper abrasions sometimes penetrate the dermis and may be difficult to differentiate from a laceration. These wounds must be thoroughly cleaned before repairing or applying a dressing. The wound should be

J.E. Herrera and G. Cooper (eds.), *Essential Sports Medicine,*
doi: 10.1007/978-1-59745-414-8, © Humana Press 2008

scrubbed clean with a mild soap followed by copious irrigation with normal saline or a balanced salt solution (e.g., Ringer's lactate solution). Materials such as harsh soaps, iodophors, or alcohol should not be used because these materials are cytotoxic and may delay healing. The wound may bleed after cleansing and débridement. Applying an antibiotic ointment and covering it with a sterile dressing is recommended. Athletes should be instructed on basic wound care and may return to competition if they can compete safely. Open wounds should be covered before returning to contact sports.

A laceration is a full thickness wound of the skin that may result from contact with sharp objects or compression of the skin against the bone with a blunt object. Lacerations are among the most common sports injuries. Significant bleeding may be present if vessels were severed. On-site treatment goals include cleaning and obtaining hemostasis. Direct pressure will assist in controlling the bleeding and will prevent hematoma formation, which predisposes to infection, wound breakdown, and scarring. Wounds may be closed primarily up to 48 hours following injury. Delayed primary wound closure may be indicated if there is facial bone fracture, extensive facial edema, or hematoma. Open treatment of some facial bone fractures can be accessed through the laceration, which will be closed at the time of fracture repair.

Treatment of tongue lacerations varies depending upon their size, location, and amount of hemorrhage. Small posterior lacerations without significant bleeding may go untreated, but larger lacerations likely to cause annoying scarring or that need hemorrhage control should be sutured. Tongue lacerations may need to be explored for foreign bodies, including tooth fragments.

Wounds that have been contaminated by any foreign material must be thoroughly examined and cleaned. Lacerations that involve the lip vermillion border, facial nerve deficits, ear or nose cartilage, eyebrow, eyelid, and significant depth are at risk for poor cosmetic or functional outcomes and need a referral for appropriate care. Early treatment of soft tissue injuries will minimize scarring and decrease potentially adverse psychological effects. A pulsive-type irrigating device can help remove debris or other loose material. Tetanus prophylaxis should be instituted with contaminated wounds. Although infection of uncomplicated head and neck soft tissue injuries is rare, some may need antibiotic prophylaxis. Lacerations that are hemostatic and appropriately covered may allow for return to play. Athletes who require complex laceration repairs generally can not return to play. Wound strength gradually increases with healing. Wound strength increases to 20% by 3 weeks and to 50% by 4 weeks. At 3–6 months, a wound achieves its maximum strength, which is 70–80% of its original strength. Avulsions injuries that include the actual loss of tissue are uncommon in sports injuries. These may require staged or multiple procedures.

## 3   Facial Bone Fractures

A recent review of facial fractures sustained during sports participation notes that in the medical literature, sporting activities account for 3–29% of facial injuries and 10–42% of all facial fractures. Sports that present the highest risk are those that involve small objects that are propelled at high velocity, such as baseball, softball, hockey, lacrosse, jai alai, and racquetball, and those with high levels of physical contact and collision, such as football, basketball, rugby, hockey, martial arts, and boxing.

Nearly 75% of facial fractures occur in the mandible, zygoma, and nose. Sports participation is the most common cause of mandibular fractures (31.5%), followed closely by motor vehicle accidents (27.2%). A recent study of facial fractures sustained during recreational baseball and softball demonstrated that the zygoma or zygomatic arch was the most common fracture, followed by temporoparietal skull fractures and orbital blowout fractures. There is some evidence to indicate that the nasal bones are the most commonly fractured bones in the face; however, many of these patients do not seek medical treatment or are managed in the outpatient setting, therefore the statistics may not be completely accurate. As is true for all injuries, an accurate history will help properly diagnose the problem.

The bones of the face are traditionally divided into thirds. The upper third includes the frontal bone. The middle third or midface includes the maxilla, zygoma, lacrimal, nasal, palatine, inferior nasal concha, and vomer bones. The lower third includes the mandible with its temporomandibular joint.

## 3.1   Upper Third

The frontal bone forms the anterior portion of the cranium, houses the frontal sinuses, and forms the roof of the ethmoid sinuses, nose, and orbit. The inferior surface of the frontal bone forms the concave surface of the orbital roof and the anterior nasal roof. The frontal bone articulates with the zygoma laterally and the maxilla and nasal bones medially.

## 3.2   Midface

The maxilla, which forms the upper jaw is a paired bone, fused at the midline, and susceptible to facial trauma and fracture. It is the central focus of the middle third of the face. The zygomatic process of the maxilla arises from the anterolateral corner of the maxilla and articulates laterally with the zygoma. Medial to the zygomatic arch, the nasal bones articulate with the frontal bone superiorly and with each other in the midline. The inferior portions of the nasal bones are thin and are the most common area where fractures occur.

René Le Fort first described fractures of the maxillary region in 1901. Le Fort I fractures involve a transverse fracture of the maxilla above the level of root apices and through the floor of the nasal cavity. Le Fort II (pyramidal) fractures pass through the frontal-nasal articulation, lacrimal bones, floor of the orbit, lateral wall of the maxilla, and through the pterygomaxillary buttress. Le Fort III injuries, also known as craniofacial dysjunction, require significant force and usually are caused by motor vehicle or motorcycle accidents and result in the midface being separated from the cranial base. They are a relatively uncommon sports injury. They may be associated with a high-velocity shearing force injury such as from a hockey puck, baseball pitch, or baseball bat.

Fractures of the zygomaticomaxillary complex (ZMC) are another common midface injury. This complex plays a key role in structure, function, and aesthetic appearance of the midface. It provides normal cheek contour and separates the orbital contents from the temporal fossa and the maxillary sinus. The ZMC forms the inferolateral orbit and provides lateral globe support. Interruption of the orbital floor often causes diplopia. The zygomatic arch is the insertion site for the masseter muscle, the most important muscle of mastication. Zygomatic complex fractures are the second most common type of facial fracture. Commonly, a fracture involves a central depression of the arch with loss of the cheek prominence. Isolated arch fractures are less common. Physical examination of the ZMC includes palpating the zygomatic arch and buttress regions. The athlete may report a forceful blow to the cheek with a bat or an elbow. The most common signs and symptoms associated with ZMC fractures are pain, edema, asymmetry, ecchymosis, and subconjunctival hemorrhage. Complaints often include numbness in the distribution of the infraorbital nerve and trismus. Other symptoms include diplopia and malocclusion. Physical findings include facial distortion in the form of an elongated face, a mobile maxilla, or midface instability. Examination of the midface is performed using the thumb and index finger. Simultaneously palpate the buccal fold region to rule out Le Fort I injuries. The nasofrontal region should be palpated to rule out Le Fort II or III maxillary fractures. Manipulation of the maxilla should provoke instability if fractures are present. Some fractures may cause significant disruption of the orbital floor and result in intraocular injury. Injuries resulting in significant disruption of the bony orbit require an ophthalmological evaluation.

Midface fractures are very difficult to assess with plane radiography and are now diagnosed using facial CT scans with coronal and axial cuts. Surgical intervention is indicated in patients with injuries that will result in a significant cosmetic or functional deformity. Open reduction and internal fixation to restore normal contour is the surgical standard of care. Prophylactic antibiotics are warranted if the fracture extends through the tooth-bearing region or through the nasal or sinus mucosa.

Nasal bone fractures are very common sports injuries. The central protuberant position on the face predisposes these bones to injury. Fractures can be classified as open or closed, depending on the integrity of the mucosa. The direction of the force to the nose determines the type of fracture. Inferior blows to the lower two thirds of the nose are likely to cause septal fractures and dislocations, while lateral blows often displace the nasal bone. Sports-related nasal injuries are usually isolated and rarely constitute an emergency. Intense frontal traumas can result in extensive fractures of the nasoethmoidal complex and can cause a depressed, widened nasal bridge. These patients often have significant midfacial injury and may have cerebrospinal fluid leakage.

Clinical presentation of nasal fractures can include epistaxis, nasal deformity, nasal airway obstruction, and infraorbital ecchymosis. Indications for repair of nasal fractures include compromised function, cosmetic deformity, and the presence of postinjury complications. Reduction of a deviated septum or uncomplicated fractures may be attempted in the field immediately after injury by using gentle hand pressure. Nasal splinting is often needed to prevent dislocation of the reduced fracture.

Surgical repair is best performed early, within hours following the injury, or in 10–14 days once the swelling and edema has resolved. Any open wounds require antibiotics.

Epistaxis, another common sports related injury, usually originates from the Kiesselbach's plexus, or the anterior septum. Packing the nasal aperture with gauze can control most anterior nosebleeds. Persistent bleeding may indicate a complex fracture that requires direct visualization with adequate lighting and instrumentation.

Athletes can return to play if hemostasis is obtained. Protective devices should be worn during contact sports for at least 4 weeks after injury.

Medical management of midface fractures includes a soft diet, analgesia, and close follow-up care. The ultimate goal in treating these midface fractures is to obtain an accurate stable reduction while minimizing external scars and functional deformity. Surgical intervention is either immediate before the onset of significant edema or several days after the injury when most of the tissue edema has resolved and any residual deformity can be appreciated more readily.

## 3.3  Lower Face

The mandible is a U-shaped bone, composed of the body, two rami, and their articulating temporomandibular joints. It is the only mobile bone of the facial skeleton, and proper motion is essential for adequate mastication.

Fractures of the mandible are common. These fractures can involve any region of the body, ramus, condyle, or joint. The direction and magnitude of the force influence the sites of the fracture and the amount and direction of bone displacement. Complicated mandible fractures may cause significant swelling and airway embarrassment. A literature review indicates the risk of mandibular fractures is highest during rugby and soccer but occurs in all contact sports. When fractures pass through dentate areas, the patients usually report malocclusion in addition to jaw pain or lip and chin numbness. Palpation of the oral and facial soft tissues often reveals mobility of bony segments. Malocclusion and eccentric movements during attempted function are typical findings for mandibular fractures. Mandibular fractures are optimally diagnosed by dental panoramic x-rays. Plane films, including right and left lateral obliques and posteroanterior or CT scanning, can also be used. Mandibular fractures that are treated earlier heal better with fewer complications.

Mandibular fractures can be treated by closed reduction with maxillomandibular fixation (MMF) utilizing interdental wiring, or open reduction and bony fixation with small plates and screws. Goals of treatment should include anatomical stabilization of fracture segments and restoration of premorbid occlusion. Ideally, treatment should be instituted within 3 days. Open reduction allows for direct evaluation of the mandibular segments and the best possible anatomic reduction.

Return to play is based upon the type and severity of the injury as well as the treatment modality employed.

The temporomandibular joint (TMJ) is a freely movable synovial joint located between the glenoid fossa of the temporal bone and the head of the mandibular condyle below. The articular surfaces of the joint and the condyle are covered by avascular fibrocartilage and are unlike most joint surfaces, which are covered by hyaline cartilage. A fibrocartilaginous disc is interposed between the joint surfaces.

Most condylar fractures arise from blunt trauma to the anterior mandible. Posterior movement of the mandible within the glenoid fossa of the TMJ is limited, resulting in fractures. The condylar fragment can dislocate out of the fossa, usually anteriorly. Symmetrical impact will result in bilateral fractures and unilateral impact will cause contralateral condylar fractures.

On physical exam, a unilateral condylar fracture results in deviation of the jaw upon opening toward the side of the fracture. Bilateral fractures produce an anterior open bite with little or no chin deviation. Radiological imaging in two planes is required. Minimally displaced fractures are usually treated by closed reduction with maxillomandibular fixation, early mobilization, and physical therapy. Displaced fractures may have to be treated by open reduction with internal fixation. Bilateral fractures usually require open reduction. Early mobilization will reduce the development of soft tissue scarring and ankylosis. Return to play is determined by the type of injury and treatment modality employed.

Temporomandibular joint dislocation is caused by lateral forces. It may be unilateral or bilateral. Joint reduction can often be accomplished shortly after the injury without sedation, before severe facial edema and muscle spasm develop. With the patient sitting, the physician stands in front of the patient and places thumbs inside the mouth, lateral to the teeth, and as far posteriorly as possible. Downward and posterior traction will reduce the dislocation.

The clinician is reminded that any significant maxillofacial injury can be accompanied by cervical spine injury. The C-spine should always be assessed clinically and radiologically if indicated, and injuries here should be ruled out prior to manipulation of the neck.

## 4 Dental Injuries

Participation in contact sports such as hockey, boxing, soccer, baseball, football, and wrestling can result in dental trauma. In the United States, the National Youth Sports Foundation estimates that more than 5 million teeth will be avulsed in sporting events each year. The Centers for Disease Control and Prevention in 2001 estimated that approximately one third of all dental injuries in the United States are sports related. After trauma, the dentition should be examined for fractures and mobility. Injuries to the teeth and supporting structures should be treated emergently.

The time interval from injury to treatment is important to successfully retain the teeth. Missing teeth must be accounted for during examination of the oral cavity since aspiration must be ruled out.

## 4.1   Anatomy

Teeth are found in individual sockets within the maxillary and mandibular bone. Each tooth has a root and crown. The root contains the vascular pulp; the blood and nerve supply the tooth, and is connected to the socket by a periodontal ligament. The crown is the enamel shell that protects the inner layer of yellowish soft dentin and part of the pulp that extends into the crown. The gingival tissue overlies the mandible and maxilla and helps seal the tooth into the socket.

Dental injuries include fractures, luxation, avulsion, and other associated maxillofacial trauma. A fracture typically disrupts the enamel and may involve the dentin or pulp. They are usually caused by a direct blow to the tooth or indirect blow transmitted through the jaw. Fractures can affect the root, crown, or both. Fractures can be classified into simple, where they involve only the enamel; or complex, including pulp involvement. Pulp involvement can be identified by bleeding pink or red dot in the center of the dentin. Pulp exposure can be very painful. Dental injuries that involve the root and pulp are considered severe and require dental evaluation and care. Root canal therapy and crown repair are usually possible.

Luxation is the displacement of a tooth laterally, extruded or intruded. A laterally luxated tooth will be displaced anterior or posterior to the adjacent teeth. An extruded tooth will appear longer than adjacent teeth and an intruded tooth will appear shorter than the adjacent teeth. Any significant displacement typically disrupts the bony socket and tears the periodontal ligament. All luxated teeth should be repositioned immediately if they are unstable. Panoramic radiographs are recommended for all trauma-induced loose teeth to rule out unsuspected underlying bony injury.

Tooth avulsion is total separation of the tooth from the socket. This injury involves a complete tear of the periodontal ligaments. Minimizing the time from the injury to reimplantation is crucial to tooth survival. The tooth must be found and protected in order to increase the chance of successful healing. If the athlete is alert, the tooth should be immediately repositioned into its socket. If the tooth cannot be repositioned, it should be stored in a moist environment for transfer such as in a "Save-a-Tooth" kit, cold milk, cold normal saline solution in the athlete's cheek or under the tongue. Primary or "baby teeth" do not need to be reimplanted.

Studies published in both the USA and UK show how protective devices have decreased the number of dental injuries. Mouth protectors have proved to be an effective means of reducing the degree and incidence of dental trauma associated with contact sports. Mouth guards are commonly used in boxing; but other sports have been reluctant to adopt them. The incidence of dental and oral soft tissue injuries decreases to less than 1% when mouthguards are mandatory for football players. Conversely, when basketball players do not wear mouthguards, more than one fourth of the injuries involve the teeth, tongue, and lips. Mouthguards protect the teeth, reduce oral lacerations and contusions, and are thought to decrease the risk of facial fractures. These devices can be store bought, mouth-formed, or custom made by a dentist. The stock mouth guard comes in set sizes and is the least protective and cheapest. They are loose fitting and are held in place by keeping the teeth together and jaw closed. The mouth-formed is the most commonly worn and provides mediocre support. The athletes tend to bite down on the thick lining, reducing the cushioning of the teeth and rendering it ineffective. Custom made mouthguards are made by a dentist to perfectly fit the athlete's mouth. The athlete can breathe, and properly articulate while wearing the mouthguard. Professionally made mouthguards clearly provide the best protection for the athlete.

Decisions about returning to play depend upon the dental injury sustained. Injuries to the enamel only, or through the enamel and dentin can allow an athlete to return immediately if the soft tissue bleeding is controlled and a properly fitted mouthguard is being worn. The athlete should see a dentist within 48 hours. Immediate return to play is not recommended if the teeth are significantly displaced or intraoral laceration is not hemostatic. The athlete can consider return to play after a luxated tooth has been repositioned properly, but should seek dental consultation as soon as possible. Athletes with avulsions should not return to play and should seek dental consultation immediately.

Athletes need to regain their confidence in returning to play. An athlete who has physically recovered may not be mentally recovered from the trauma of the injury and, thus is at risk of further injury. This is often observed in baseball players who are hit in the face by a pitch or hit ball. Psychological recovery from facial fractures can be assessed in controlled practice situations. A consult with a sports psychologist may be necessary if difficulties linger.

Many sports have safety measures to limit the incidence of facial injuries, and attention should be paid to the rules of use. Racquetball players should always play with goggles to limit orbital blowout injuries. In hockey, face guards with helmets are required in lower levels of play but not at the professional level. Although baseball is not considered a contact sport, sliding injuries can result in ankle sprains and fractures as well as serious head injuries. In 1995, the US Consumer Product Safety Commission performed an extensive review of all baseball injuries in youth baseball players aged 5 to 14. The commission found a high incidence of head and neck injuries in youth players and estimated that approximately one third of the injuries could have been prevented with protective equipment, including helmets. The best way to decrease the number of facial injuries sustained during sports is through proper prevention.

# References

1. Amy E (2005) Oro-facial injuries in Central American and Caribbean sports games: a 20-year experience. Dental Traumatol 21:127–130
2. Bak MJ, Doerr TD (2004) Craniomaxillofacial fractures during recreational baseball and softball. J Oral Maxillofacial Surg 62:1209–1212

3. Boden BP, Tacchetti R, Mueller FO (2004) Catastrophic injuries in high school and college baseball players. Am J Sports Med 32:1189–1196

4. Booth PW, Eppley BL, Schmelzeisen R (2003) Maxillofacial trauma and esthetic facial reconstruction. Elsevier Science, Philadelphia

5. Delibasi C, Yamazawa M, Nomura K, Iida S, Kogo M (2004) Oral Surg Oral Med Oral Pathol 97:23–27

6. Exadaktylos AK, Eggensperger NM, Eggli S, Smolka KM, Zimmerman H, Iizuka T (2004) Sports related maxillofacial injuries: the first maxillofacial trauma database in Switzerland. Br J Sports Med 38:750–753

7. Fonseca RJ, Walker RV (1991) Oral and maxillofacial trauma. WB Saunders, Philadelphia

8. Gassner R, Tuli T, Hachl O, Rudisch A, Ulmer H (2003) Cranio-maxillofacial trauma: a 10 year review of 9,543 cases with 21,067 injuries. J Craniomaxillofacial Surg 31:51–61

9. Hill CM, Burford K, Martin A, Thomas DW (1998) A one-year review of maxillofacial sports injuries treated at an accident and emergency department. Br J Oral Maxillofacial Surg 36:44–47

10. Hill CM, Crosher RF, Mason DA (1985) Dental and facial injuries following sports accidents: a study of 130 patients. Br J Oral Maxillofacial Surg 23:268–274

11. Honsik KA, Harmon KG, Rubin A (2004) Emergency treatment of dentoalveolar trauma. Phys Sportsmed 23:9

12. Iida S, Kogo M, Sugiura T, Mima T, Matsuya T (2001) Retrospective analysis of 1502 patients with facial fractures. Int J Oral Maxillofacial Surg 30:286–290

13. MacAfee KA (1994) Primary care management of maxillofacial injuries in sports. Penn Dent J 93:16–17, 25

14. Mourouzis C, Koumoura F (2005) Sports-related maxillofacial fractures: a retrospective study of 125 patients. Int J Oral Maxillofacial Surg 34:635–638

15. Porras-Reyes BH, Mustoe TA (1994) Wound healing. In: Cohen M (ed) Mastery of plastic and reconstructive surgery. Little, Brown, Boston pp. 3–13

16. Roberts WO (2000) Field care of the injured tooth. Phys Sportsmed 28:101

17. Romeo S, Hawley C, Romeo M, Romeo J (2005) Facial injuries in sports: a team physician's guide to diagnosis and treatment. Phys Sportsmed 33, 4

18. Stackhouse T, Howe WB (1998) On-site management of nasal injuries. Phys Sportsmed 26:69

# Chapter 4
# Cervical Spine Injuries

**Dorothy A. Miller and Thomas N. Bryce**

## 1  Introduction

Ten percent of the roughly 10,000 new spinal cord injuries (SCIs) sustained annually in the United States are sports related. The five most frequent sports responsible for SCI in descending order of incidence and total percentage of all SCIs are: diving (3.9%), snow skiing (0.9%), football (0.5%), surfing (0.5%), and horseback riding (0.5%). Sports-related injuries are the second most common cause, following motor vehicle accidents (MVAs), for neck-related emergency room visits. Most sports-related injuries involve soft tissue trauma such as ligament sprains, muscle strains, and soft tissue contusions. Fortunately severe cervical spine injuries are rare. However, physicians who treat sports medicine injuries are often responsible for the emergency care of such injured athletes and must know the spectrum of injuries that can occur. They must also know how to assess and manage these injuries on the field.

## 2  Anatomy of Cervical Spine

Compared with the relatively rigid thoracic spine and moderately flexible lumbar spine, the cervical spine is the most flexible of the three allowing significant range of motion (ROM) in all planes at the cost of relative stability, especially when the structures of the neck are stressed. The region relies heavily on ligaments and other soft tissue structures to maintain physiological ROM. The cervical spine is composed of seven vertebrae. The occipital-atlantal and C1-C2 joints together account for 34% of the available cervical flexion and extension, whereas 54% of the total cervical rotation takes place at C1-C2. Motion at this these joints, however, accounts for only 10% of lateral bending. The greatest cervical flexion and extension takes place at C5-C6 and C6-C7, whereas the greatest side bending occurs at C2-C3 and C3-C4 with relatively less motion in all planes occurring at the lowest cervical levels. Excessive pathological neck mobility is kept in check by both static and dynamic stabilizers. Static stabilizers include the following structures: the anterior longitudinal ligament (ALL), posterior longitudinal ligament (PLL), intervertebral disc, ligamentum flavum, facet capsules, interspinous ligaments, and

J.E. Herrera and G. Cooper (eds.), *Essential Sports Medicine,*
doi: 10.1007/978-1-59745-414-8, © Humana Press 2008

supraspinous ligament. Of these, the posterior structures, PLL, ligamentum flavum, facet capsules, interspinous ligaments, and supraspinous ligament contribute more to stability in flexion; whereas the anterior ligaments, ALL, and discs contribute more to stability on extension. The major muscles that act as dynamic stabilizers of the cervical spine controlling the degree and speed of movement of the spine are the paraspinals, trapezius, sternocleidomastoid, and lateral strap muscles.

# 3   Stable Cervical Spine Injuries

## 3.1   Acute Cervical Strain Syndrome

### 3.1.1   Mechanism of Injury

Acute cervical strains are muscular stretch injuries that occur most commonly at the musculotendinous junction and less commonly within the muscle body itself. They are induced by mechanical overloading of the musculotendinous tissue and can often result in a tearing of the muscle or tendon. The most common muscles affected are the trapezius, sternocleidomastoids, erector spine, scalenes, levator scapulae, and rhomboids. The strained muscle overstretches while eccentrically contracting. Cervical facet mechanoreceptors provide proprioceptive feedback to neck stabilizer muscles and are thought to help instigate protective contraction of these structures at the time of strain.

### 3.1.2   Clinical Presentation and Diagnosis

The athlete's first complaint after experiencing a cervical strain is local pain, tenderness, and/or weakness in the neck. The athlete is able to maintain full ROM of the cervical spine immediately after injury. The athlete complains of muscle pain that peaks several hours postinjury. However, mild strains may not manifest symptomatically until the following morning, at which time muscle soreness, swelling, and mild limitation in ROM may occur. Pain is typically exacerbated by muscle stretch. The extent of tissue damage correlates roughly with the relative limitation in ROM, swelling, and discomfort experienced 24–48 hours postinjury. This condition often accompanies a brachial plexus injury. Athletes with painful ROM of the neck should undergo flexion/extension radiographs of the cervical spine to rule out instability and fracture.

### 3.1.3   Treatment

Treatment is symptomatic and includes anti-inflammatory medications, rest, ice, and heat after 24 hours. For more severe strains, a soft foam cervical orthosis may be prescribed for use until the initial muscle spasm has passed, most often 7–10 days.

At this time the soft cervical orthosis can be removed and gentle active ROM initiated. Cervical isometric neck strengthening exercises may also be started. With continued clinical improvement, functional and sports-specific exercises are introduced. Although commonly prescribed, the use of a soft foam cervical orthosis is controversial. In 2000 and 2003, Rosenfeld et al. published two articles that compared active neck exercises without cervical orthosis with a protocol involving rest, soft collar use, and self-mobilization; these studies were performed in persons who had suffered whiplash injuries. The authors found that the patients whose clinical course did not involve orthosis use had less pain and fewer lost days from work.

### 3.1.4   Return to Play

The athlete may return to play after he or she has regained preinjury neck muscle strength, full cervical ROM, and is asymptomatic. Returning early may result in repeated cervical strains and the risk of more serious future cervical spine injury. After returning to sport, performance of a regular cervical exercise program may help prevent further injury.

## 3.2   Acute Cervical Sprain

### 3.2.1   Mechanism of Injury

Acute cervical sprains are ligamentous stretch injuries resulting from distraction injuries to the cervical spine's ligaments and capsular structures. Hyperextension of neck with concomitant compression can produce facet joint and peri-facet joint soft tissue trauma. Numerous tears in the fascia can occur with rupture of small vessels within the soft tissues of the neck, which may ultimately result in fibrous tissue contraction and possible limitation in neck ROM. The joints of Luschka and their capsular ligaments are extremely susceptible to sprain. Acute cervical sprains may be accompanied by traumatic compression neuropathies.

### 3.2.2   Clinical Presentation and Diagnosis

Pain is generally limited to the neck, upper arm, or area between the scapulae. Hyperesthesias may be present from a concomitant compression neuropathy. Cervical extension ROM is often decreased. Athletes with persistent painful ROM of the neck should undergo static and flexion/extension radiographs of the cervical spine to rule out instability and fracture. An MRI of the cervical spine should be performed if there are any persistent neurological changes detected on physical exam.

### 3.2.3  Treatment

The treatment is identical to that for cervical strain.

### 3.2.4  Return to Play

The return to play criteria are identical to that for cervical strain.

## 3.3  Acute Cervical Disc Herniation

### 3.3.1  Mechanism of Injury

An acute cervical disc herniation most often occurs as a result of excessive neck flexion. The annulus of the intervertebral disc can tear with extrusion of the nucleus pulposus to tissues outside the disc. The nucleus pulposus contains proinflammatory cytokines, most notably TNF-α that can chemically irritate surrounding tissue, in addition to physically compressing neighboring structures. The ligamentous architecture of the cervical spine dictates that the most common orientation of herniation is posterior-lateral.

### 3.3.2  Clinical Presentation

Acute cervical disc herniation usually occurs in older athletes. However, high-performance wrestlers and football players are at especially high risk. Compression of a particular nerve root by a herniated nucleus pulposus (HNP) or chemical irritation of that nerve by this material may cause radicular symptoms with localized cervical pain. Such patients are often most comfortable with the neck in a neutral or slightly hyperextended posture; symptoms are often relieved by gentle traction. Symptoms are often reproduced by a positive Spurling's test. In this test, the patient's head is passively extended and laterally rotated to the side of symptoms. Gentle axial compression is then applied by the examiner. Reproduction of symptoms indicates a positive test.

### 3.3.3  Diagnosis

Athletes with any persistent radicular symptoms or evidence of myelopathy should undergo an MRI of the cervical spine to evaluate for nerve root or spinal cord compression.

### 3.3.4   Treatment

If there is evidence of cord compression with myelopathy, i.e., tetraplegia, emergent decompression is indicated; this is accomplished most often through an anterior surgical approach and usually includes removal of the offending disc and fusion of the adjacent vertebral bodies. If the patient is nonmyelopathic, then rest, NSAIDs, immobilization, cervical traction, and potentially fluoroscopically guided epidural steroid injections are indicated. In the rare event that an injured athlete with an extremely laterally oriented cervical HNP presents with only arm pain and there is no cord compression, the athlete may benefit from a less invasive microforaminotomy instead of discectomy and fusion. This is a procedure in which the affected foramen is surgically widened to relieve pressure on the peripheral nerve being compressed by the HNP.

### 3.3.5   Return to Play

Absolute contraindications to returning to contact sports include the following: a three-level cervical spine fusion and symptomatic cervical disc herniation. Relative contraindications include a healed and stable two-level subaxial cervical fusion. Athletes who have undergone fusion at one to two levels of the lower cervical spine are at a lower risk for further injury when returning to play than those undergoing instrumentation at higher levels as a fusion structure present in the distal cervical spine is able to absorb more force than one more proximally oriented. Players who have undergone a one-level subaxial fusion without instrumentation as well as those status-post single or multilevel posterior microlaminoforaminotomies have no contraindication to returning to contact sports participation. Observing these caveats, athletes may return to sport once asymptomatic with normal cervical spine stabilizing muscle strength and expected cervical spine mobility.

## 3.4   Transient Brachial Plexopathy and Radiculopathy

### 3.4.1   Mechanism of Injury

Transient brachial plexopathies and radiculopathies, commonly referred to as "stingers" or "burners" result from trauma to the brachial plexus or nerve roots. The mechanism of injury is traction to these neurological structures that occur when the head is forcibly laterally tilted and extended as the contralateral shoulder is depressed. They often occur at the time of a block or tackle in football. As many as 65% of collegiate football players are diagnosed with at least one career stinger; most of these players are defensive linemen. Other etiologies include compression of nerve roots in their foramina during forced lateral neck bending or a direct blow to the brachial plexus at Erb's point. Most transient brachial plexopathies affect the upper trunk of the brachial plexus. There is a higher incidence of transient brachial plexopathies and radiculopathies in athletes with cervical spinal stenosis. MRI evaluation of athletes with recurrent events showed that 53% had cervical spinal stenosis and 87% had degenerative disc disease. The Torg ratio is a measure of congenital spinal stenosis that has been found to correlate with transient brachial plexopathy and radiculopathy incidence; the Torg ratio is determined by drawing an AP diameter line is drawn connecting the midpoint of the posterior vertebral body line to the spinothalaminar line. This value is then divided by the width of the vertebral body from the anterior to posterior-most parts. In a study by Meyer et al, college athletes with a Torg ratio of <0.8 were three times more likely to sustain transient brachial plexopathy and radiculopathy with cervical spine injuries involving neck compression and extension than those with a Torg ratio >0.8.

### 3.4.2   Clinical Presentation and Diagnosis

Transient brachial plexopathies and radiculopathies are usually always unilateral. Athletes demonstrate the inability to move the upper extremity immediately following a high-energy collision. The athlete may complain of a burning pain and/or numbness in the affected limb. As the upper trunk of the brachial plexus is the most commonly affected, the deltoid (C5), biceps (C5, C6), supraspinatus (C5, C6), and infraspinatus muscles (C5, C6) are most often impaired. Affected athletes have impaired shoulder abduction, external rotation, and arm flexion that may be delayed relative to their sensory symptoms. Symptoms usually resolve within minutes of injury. Affected athletes usually hold their necks in a slightly flexed position to relieve pressure of the damaged nerve root in its foramen. Positive Spurling's maneuver may be found in up to 70% of affected athletes. Athletes with any persistent radicular symptoms or evidence of myelopathy should undergo an MRI of the cervical spine to evaluate for nerve root or spinal cord compression. If persistent symptoms are referable to the brachial plexus, an MRI of the brachial plexus is warranted. Electromyography may be useful for defining the extent of the injury and may help define prognosis in incidences in which signs and symptoms have persisted for more than 2 weeks.

### 3.4.3   Treatment

The management of transient brachial plexopathies and radiculopathies is supportive. Athletes should be restricted from play until asymptomatic. If there is significant weakness of the extremity, support of the affected arm and shoulder with a sling is indicated. Oral analgesic and anti-inflammatory medications can decrease pain. Ice and heat after 24 hours are useful adjuncts. If symptoms are persistent and no treatable cord, plexus, or spinal cord compression is identified on imaging, prescription of a formal therapy program with a goal of regaining normal ROM of the cervical spine and the affected limb joints and normal strength of the cervical spine stabilizing musculature and affected limb muscles is warranted. It should be noted that failure to regain full cervical spine ROM may contribute to continued root irritation if this is the cause of the problem.

### 3.4.4 Return to Play

If the athlete has two transient brachial plexopathies or radiculopathies within a single season or spread out over several seasons, then the athlete has no restriction on returning to sports. The athlete can return to play the same day as long as he or she demonstrates full and pain free cervical spine ROM and upper extremity strength. Relative contraindications to return to play in the future include the following: symptoms lasting more than 24 hours, and three or more previous transient brachial plexopathies or radiculopathies with full pain-free cervical ROM and neck strength. Continued cervical neck discomfort with impaired ROM, or any evidence of neurological deficit represent absolute contraindications to play; the athlete should not be allowed to return to play if he or she has evidence of cervical disc herniation or cervical instability. If the athlete has had one or two prior brachial plexopathies or radiculopathies each lasting <24 hours and the current brachial plexopathy or radiculopathy does not resolve while the player is sitting out that game, then the athlete must undergo imaging. The goal of radiographic or MRI evaluation is to find an underlying anatomical lesion predisposing the athlete to repeated injury or to find a potentially treatable cause of persistent signs and symptoms.

## 3.5 Cervical Spinous Process Fracture

### 3.5.1 Mechanism of Injury

Spinous process fractures most often occur at the lower cervical and upper thoracic levels and are often an isolated bony finding. When it affects C7, it is called clay shoveler's fracture. Three mechanisms of injury have been described: avulsion of the spinous process following strong contraction of trapezius and rhomboid, direct hit to the spinous process, and spinous process avulsion by intraspinous and supraspinous ligaments during forced c-spine hyperextension or hyperflexion. This latter mechanism occurs only with high-velocity trauma such as in football or MVA.

### 3.5.2 Treatment

A soft cervical orthosis can be prescribed to help limit ROM and the resultant pain, which can arise from movement. ROM should not be advised until at least 4–6 weeks after injury to allow fracture healing. Flexion and extension radiographs should be performed at that time to reassess stability.

### 3.5.3 Return to Play

The player can return to play if asymptomatic and there is no sagittal plane kyphotic deformity evidenced on follow-up lateral radiographs of the cervical spine.

## 4 Unstable Cervical Spine Injuries

Cervical instability can result from bony and/or ligamentous damage. White and Johnson et al. defined cervical instability as the inability of the neck to support the head while protecting the spinal cord or its nerve roots from disruption by the cervical column. In contact sports, instability is most often induced by axial compression with neck flexion. White determined that the adult cervical spine is unstable when at least one of the following criteria are met: all anterior or posterior elements are destroyed or otherwise rendered unable to function; >3.5 mm of horizontal vertebral subluxation is present on lateral radiographs (resting or flexion/extension); or 11 degrees or more of angular displacement exists between adjacent vertebrae as measured on either resting or flexion/extension radiographs. When assessing cervical stability, radiographs must be taken from the occiput to the C7-T1 junction. Several additional radiological abnormalities may indicate cervical instability, including vertebral subluxation, vertebral compression fractures, and loss of cervical lordosis. Loss of cervical lordosis in itself is not a sign of instability, but it may indicate masking of underlying instability by paracervical muscle spasm. In contrast, this muscle spasm causing loss of cervical lordosis may just be the body's attempt to minimize movement in a painful but not necessarily unstable area after trauma.

The most common cause of catastrophic cervical spine trauma is the development of an unstable cervical fracture. Mechanistically, axial force application to the top of the head decelerates the head and thereby positions the cervical spine to absorb much of the force of the oncoming body. The position of the neck at the time of impact in addition to the force of impact largely determines the type and extent of injury sustained. The physiological position of the cervical spine is in neutral with a slight lordotic posture. In this position, the posterior elements are engaged in such a way that maximizes the cervical spine's absorption of axial compressive force. When flexed, the above mentioned lordosis decreases and the cervical spine is much more vulnerable to serious injury on axial compression. The two most common mechanisms of injury causing catastrophic cervical spinal column injuries in contact sports are compression-flexion and straight axial compression. Compression-flexion forces cause fracture of the anterior column. Flexion teardrops fractures result from hyperflexion of the subaxial cervical spine (C3-C7) and are characterized by retropulsion of the fractured vertebral body into the spinal canal. Flexion teardrop fractures are associated with posterior facet and ligamentous disruption and often accompany an anterior cord syndrome. Sometimes these fractures are associated with complete SCI. Central cord syndrome results when the spinal cord is compressed between the vertebral body and the ligamentum flavum and/or hypertrophied facet joints; central cord syndrome is seen only in cervical spine injury and is characterized by sacral sensory sparing and more pronounced weakness in the arms relative to the legs.

A second type of compression injury results from direct vertical compression and is called a "burst fracture." In this scenario, the intradiscal pressure increases to such a level that the vertebral body shatters. In the process, pieces of vertebral body bone may be forced backward into the canal, thereby compressing the cord. These fractures usually include at least two columns and are generally unstable and often are associated with SCI.. The lower part of the cervical spine is fractured or dislocated most frequently. Fractures and dislocations in the upper cervical spine are rare; such injuries are less apt to compress the cord because the relative canal size the larger in the upper cervical spine compared with the lower. The athlete's neurological deficits may indicate complete or incomplete cord injury. In athletics, central cord syndrome is the most common injury pattern followed by anterior cord syndrome.

## *4.1 Treatment*

Treatment of unstable cervical spine fractures is usually surgical.

## *4.2 Return to Play*

The presence of cervical spinal cord abnormality on MRI is an absolute contraindication to returning participation in contact sports. Torg et al. detailed the following comprehensive return to play criteria for unstable cervical fractures as described in this paragraph. Athletes with the following entities have no contraindication to returning to sports participation: status-post one level anterior cervical discectomy fusion (ACDF) without pain or neurological deficit, a healed and stable nondisplaced cervical fracture with no sagittal malalignment, and a one-level cervical fusion with full ROM and no evidence of instability, cervical disc disease, or other cervical degeneration. Relative contraindications include a healed two level fusion, prior upper cervical spine fracture, and healed one level fusion with lateral mass fixation. Absolute contraindications include the following: three level cervical fusion, status-post cervical laminectomy, history of C1-C2 cervical fusion, acute posterior element or cervical body fracture regardless of ligamentous involvement, healed subaxial spine fracture with residual kyphosis, or radiological evidence of distraction-extension on radiographic study.

## *4.3   Cervical Cord Neurapraxia with Transient Tetraplegia*

Transient tetraplegia most often results after an impact forcing the cervical spine into hyperextension, hyperflexion, or axial loading. Affected athletes experience tetraplegic symptoms of relatively short duration that include dysesthesias, and/or weakness in both arms, both legs, or all four extremities. Individuals do not generally complain of neck pain. The clinical symptoms last for as short as 10–15 minutes and as long as 48 hours. The patient regains full function and ROM and radiographs show no evidence of fracture, but these players often have cervical canal stenosis. In individuals with a narrowed canal in the AP diameter, the pathophysiology is thought to be as follows. Hyperextension or hyperflexion of the cervical spine causes further narrowing of the canal with compression of the cord against adjacent bony or ligamentous structures. Torg et al. found the incidence of transient cervical cord neurapraxia with transient tetraplegia to be 7 per 10,000 football athletes.

### 4.3.1   Return to Play

In addition to cervical stenosis, other pre-existing cervical abnormalities associated with transient tetraplegia include congenital fusion, kyphosis, and disc protrusion or herniation. In addition to a Torg ratio of 0.8, congenital cervical spine stenosis is diagnosed radiographically when the spinal canal diameter is <14 mm; this condition is thought to increase an athlete's risk of developing cervical spinal cord trauma. Absolute contraindications to returning to play include more than two episodes of transient tetraplegia. One prior episode of transient tetraplegia injury represents a relative contraindication to returning to play. An athlete may be allowed to play again if he or she has regained full strength and painless ROM in the neck. Mild-to-moderate spinal stenosis in the athlete who has experienced transient tetraplegia also represents a relative contraindication to play.

## References

1. Banarjee R, Palumbo MA et al. (2004) Catastrophic cervical spine injuries in the collision sport athlete, part 1: epidemiology, functional anatomy, and diagnosis. Am J Sports Med 32(4):1077–1087
2. Feinberg JH (2000) Burners and stingers. Phys Med Rehab Clin North Am 11:771–784
3. Hershman EB et al. (1990) Brachial plexus injuries. Clin Sports Med 9:311
4. Jackson AB et al. (2004) A demographic pofile of new traumatic spinal cord injuries: change and stability over 30 years. Arch Phys Med Rehab 5(85):1740
5. Jarvinen TA et al. (2000) Muscle strain injuries. Curr Opin Rheumatol 12:155–161
6. Levitz, CL et al. (1997) The pathomechanics of chronic, recurrent cervical nerve root neurapraxia: the chronic burner syndrome. Am J Sports Med (25):73–76
7. Maroon JC et al. (1996) Athletes with cervical spine injury. Spine 32(19):2294–2299

8. Meyer PR Jr, Heim S (1989) Surgical stabilization of the cervical spine. In: Meyer PR Jr (ed) Surgery of spine trauma. Churchill Livingstone, New York, 397–423

9. Meyer SA et al. (1994) Cervical spinal stenosis and stingers in collegiate football players. Am J Sports Med (22):158–166

10. Mundt DJ et al. (1993) An epidemiologic study of sports and weight lifting as possible risk factors for herniated lumbar and cervical discs. The Northeast Collaborative Group on low back pain. Am J Sports Med 21(6):854–860

11. Reid DC et al. (1989) Spine fractures in winter sports. Sports Med 7(6):393–399

12. Rosenfeld M, Gunnarsson R, Borenstein P (2000) Early intervention in whiplash-associated disorders: a comparison of two treatment protocols. Spine 25(14):1782–1787

13. Rosenfeld M, Seferiadis A, Carlsson J, Gunnarsson R (2003) Active intervention in patients with whiplash-associated disorders improves long-term prognosis: a randomized controlled clinical trial. Spine 28(22):2491–2498

14. Sallis RE et al. (1992) Burners: offensive strategy in an underreported injury. Phys Sportsmed 20:47–55

15. Torg JS, Guille JT et al. (2002) Injuries to the cervical spine in American football players. J Bone Joint Surg North Am (84):112–122

16. Torg JS et al. (1997) Suggested management guidelines for participation in collision activities with congenital, developmental, or post-injury lesions involving the cervical spine. Med Sci Sports Exerc (29):S256–272

17. Versteegem GJ et al. (1998) Neck sprain not arising from car accident: a retrospective study covering 25 years. Eur Spine J 7(3):201–205

18. Weinberg J et al. (2003) Etiology, treatment, and prevention of athletic "stingers." Clin Sport Med 21:493–500

19. White A, Johnson R, et al. (1975) Biomechanical analysis of clinical stability of the cervical spine. Clin Orthop Relat Res (109):85–97

20. White AA, Johnson RM, Panjabi MM, Southwick WO (1975) Biomechanical Analysis of chemical stability in the cervical spine. Clin Orthop Relat Res (109):85–96

21. White AA, Panjabe MM (1990) Clinical biomechanics of the spine. JB Lippincott, Philadelphia

22. Zmurko MG et al. (2003) Cervical sprains, disc herniations, minor fractures, and other cervical injuries in the athlete. Clin Sports Med (22):513–521

# Chapter 5
# Shoulder Injuries

Necolle Morgado and Joseph E. Herrera

## 1 Introduction

Shoulder pain in athletes is very common. It can be divided into acute injuries and chronic overuse injuries. Acute injuries occur in contact sports such as football, rugby, hockey, or lacrosse, and from a sudden trauma or falls such as seen with downhill skiing, cycling, and mountain climbing. Chronic overuse injuries to the shoulder usually occur in sports that require an overhead motion of the arm such as tennis, baseball, volleyball, and swimming.

## 2 Anatomy

### 2.1 Bones

The shoulder is composed of the humerus, scapula, and clavicle. The humerus articulates with the scapula at the glenohumeral joint and the clavicle articulates with the scapula at the acromioclavicular (AC) joint.

### 2.2 Static Stabilizers

The static stabilizers of the shoulder include the ligaments and glenoid labrum. The ligaments form a capsule that contains and stabilizes the glenohumeral joint. The glenoid labrum forms a rim that provides a wider surface for the humeral head to articulate.

The AC joint is stabilized by the acromioclavicular ligament and the coracoclavicular ligament.

J.E. Herrera and G. Cooper (eds.), *Essential Sports Medicine,*
doi: 10.1007/978-1-59745-414-8, © Humana Press 2008

## 2.3  Dynamic Stabilizers

The dynamic stabilizers of the shoulder include the rotator cuff, deltoid, biceps, and pectoral muscles. The rotator cuff muscles include the supraspinatus, infraspinatus, teres minor, and subscapularis muscles. The rotator cuff acts to depress and stabilize the glenohumeral joint.

# 3  Acute Shoulder Injuries

## 3.1  Shoulder Separation

A shoulder separation, also known as an acromioclavicular (AC) separation or sprain, occurs when the ligaments that hold the clavicle to the acromion are injured. A shoulder separation occurs from a direct blow or fall on to the acromion with arm in the adducted position. It also can result from a fall on an outstretched hand or arm.

### 3.1.1  Clinical Presentation

The presentation of shoulder separation is severe pain on the anterior lateral aspect of the shoulder at the time of injury. Depending on the severity of the injury, athletes may complain of shoulder deformity from clavicle protrusion. Limited ROM may also be present, especially with active abduction and/or forward flexion of the shoulder. Athletes who weight train may complain of pain when the joint is challenged, especially with bench pressing and dips. Other complaints may include ecchymosis and swelling of the shoulder.

### 3.1.2  Diagnosis

Physical exam reveals tenderness to palpation over the AC joint. Frank deformity from superior migration of the clavicle if present makes the diagnosis obvious. If the diagnosis is not to obvious other physical exam maneuvers including the scarf test and the AC squeeze test are helpful.

- *Scarf test:* Passive adduction of the shoulder across the chest. Reproduction of pain over the AC joint with this maneuver is positive and may indicate AC sprain.
- *AC squeeze test:* The examiner places the base of the palm on the spine of the scapula and the other hand is positioned on the clavicle. With the fingers interlocked the examiners pushes or "squeezes" the palms together (Fig. 5.1). Reproduction of pain in the AC area is considered positive.

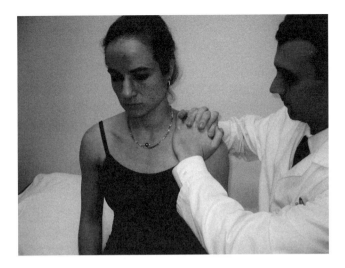

**Fig. 5.1** AC squeeze test

Diagnostic studies such as AP lateral and stress radiographs of the shoulder are important to rule out fracture and to determine the severity of injury. Stress views of the shoulder involve the use of 10–15 lb weights wrapped around the wrist. These views determines the integrity of the coracoclavicular ligament.

### 3.1.3   Grading

- *Type I:* Sprained but intact acromioclavicular and coracoclavicular ligament and no dislocation
- *Type II:* Torn acromioclavicular and intact coracoclavicular ligament and no dislocation
- *Type III:* Torn acromioclavicular and coracoclavicular ligament with possible complete dislocation and superior displacement if the clavicle
- *Type IV:* Torn acromioclavicular and coracoclavicular ligament with posterior migration of the clavicle
- *Type V:* Torn acromioclavicular and coracoclavicular ligament with superior migration and penetration of the trapezius muscle of the clavicle
- *Type VI:* Torn acromioclavicular and coracoclavicular ligament with inferior migration and penetration of the biceps muscle of the clavicle

### 3.1.4   Treatment

Acutely, the shoulder should be treated with ice, immobilization, and support with a sling. The use of analgesics and anti-inflammatories may be used as well. Further treatment will be determined by the type of injury. Grade I–III injuries can be treated with a sling or shoulder immobilizer for 2 to 4 weeks to allow the ligaments to heal. Grade IV–VI AC separation may require surgical intervention. Rehabilitation for scapular and glenohumeral stabilization should also be implemented.

### 3.1.5   Return to Play

The athlete may return to play when the athlete can demonstrate full, painless ROM and normal strength of the affected shoulder. Throwing athletes have to return to sport gradually.

## 3.2   Shoulder Dislocation

Shoulder dislocation is the complete separation of the humeral head from the articular surface of the glenoid. The glenohumeral joint is the most commonly dislocated joint in the body. Approximately 95% of shoulder dislocations occur in the anterior direction, but dislocation can also occur inferiorly, superiorly, and posteriorly. There is a high incidence of dislocation in full contact sports such as football and rugby, or sports in which violent falls may occur such as downhill skiing, mountain climbing, and cycling.

### 3.2.1   Clinical Presentation

The athlete usually experiences immediate pain after a traumatic event. When evaluating an injury athlete for shoulder dislocation, noting the position of the arm at the time of the event is important in discerning the type of injury. The most common mechanism of anterior dislocation is forced abduction and external rotation of the humerus, such as seen when a quarterback's arm is struck while in mid-throw. Other mechanisms of injury include a posterior blow to the humerus, and a fall on an outstretched arm.

### 3.2.2   Diagnosis

Physical exam usually reveals an arm that is externally rotated and slightly abducted with anterior dislocation. There is some limitation and pain with internal rotation. In posterior dislocations, the arm is usually internally rotated and adducted. There is usually a limitation in external rotation.

Diagnostic studies such as x-rays and MRIs may be useful for diagnosing fractures and soft tissue injuries.

- *X-rays AP and axillary views:* These views are useful in diagnosing glenoid fractures and/or damage to the cartilaginous surface of the humeral head known as a Hill Sachs lesion. This is usually caused by the humeral head resting on the glenoid rim during dislocation. In anterior dislocation the lesion is located on the posterior surface of the humeral head. In posterior dislocation the lesion is located on the anterior surface.
- MRIs are useful in diagnosing tissue injuries such as rotator cuff tears and labral tears. More specifically, Bankart lesions are tears of the labrum that occur after a shoulder dislocation and can be the source of future shoulder instability.

### 3.2.3 Treatment

3.2.3.1 Acute Treatment

The key to treating acute dislocation is immediate reduction of the shoulder. There are several techniques that are described for anterior dislocation.

- *Hippocratic method:* Longitudinal traction is applied to the affected arm with the examiners foot in the patient's axilla. This maneuver is accompanied with internal and external rotation.
- *Stimson method:* With the patient in the prone position, traction is provided with weights attached to the affected arm.
- *Milch maneuver:* The examiner abducts the patient's arm with one hand while applying pressure to the humeral head with the other hand. As the patient's arm is abducted, an external rotation, and traction is applied.

In posterior dislocations, the shoulder should be adducted with gentle longitudinal traction with one hand, while the other hand tries to push the humeral head anteriorly. External rotation *should not* be performed due risk of humeral head fracture.

3.2.3.2 Conservative Treatment

The affected arm is usually placed in a sling for a period ranging from 10 days to 6 weeks. Rehabilitation for the arm is started after approximately 3 weeks of immobilization. Rehabilitation usually begins with gentle ROM activities that gradually progresses to cuff strengthening and scapular stabilization exercises.

3.2.3.3 Surgical Treatment

Surgical treatment of shoulder may be indicated if the patient's occupation or sport puts him or her at risk for subsequent dislocation. Surgical treatment may include one of the following options: open repair, arthroscopic capsular repair, rotator cuff interval repair, and thermal capsulorrhaphy.

### 3.2.4   Return to Play

Athletes may return to noncontact sports that require no overhead movement in 3 months. Athletes that participate in contact sports or sports that require overhead activities may return in 4 months.

# 4   Chronic Shoulder Injuries

## 4.1   Impingement Syndrome

Impingement syndrome is also known as rotator cuff tendonitis and supraspinatus tendonitis. The causes of impingement syndrome can be classified as intrinsic or extrinsic causes. Intrinsic causes of impingement include derangement of the acromion causing damage and irritation to the supraspinatus tendon.

Extrinsic causes can be further subdivided into primary and secondary causes of impingement. Primary extrinsic impingement is due to chronic overhead movements such as that seen with baseball players, quarterbacks, swimmers, and volleyball players. Secondary extrinsic impingement is caused by muscular imbalance. This is seen in throwing athletes, more specifically those who perform overhead press while training.

### 4.1.2   Clinical Presentation

An athlete with impingement syndrome usually presents with pain in the anterior superior lateral shoulder area. They usually report pain with shoulder abduction and any other overhead movements. There may also be associated sleep disturbance due to point tenderness over the anterior-lateral aspect of the shoulder. Pain usually has a gradual onset and is associated with an increased amount of training activity, playing time, or change in athletic gear.

### 4.1.3   Diagnosis

The diagnosis of impingement syndrome can usually be made clinically. Range of motion testing usually reveals a painful arc with 45 to 120 degrees of abduction. Manual strength testing may show pain related weakness, especially with abduction, and internal and external rotation testing. The following orthopedic maneuvers also indicate impingement syndrome.

- *Neer impingement test:* This test is performed with the patient sitting or standing. The patient's arm is forcibly elevated through forward flexion while the scapula is depressed, causing compression of the greater tuberosity against the acromial surface (Fig. 5.2). Pain reflects a positive test result.
- *Hawkins impingement test:* In this test, the patient's shoulder is forward flexed to 90 degrees and internally rotated. This maneuver pushes the supraspinatus tendon against the undersurface of the acromion (Fig. 5.3). Pain is considered a positive sign.
- *Supraspinatus test "empty can test":* This test is performed by abducting the shoulder to 90 degrees, internally rotating the arm, and providing 30 degrees of horizontal abduction. The examiner resists abduction (Fig. 5.4). Pain is indicative of impingement syndrome.

Diagnostic imaging is also useful in diagnosing rotator cuff impingement. The gold standard is an MRI of the shoulder with oblique coronal and oblique sagittal planes. An increased signal on the surface of the cuff may indicate tendonitis or a partial tear.

### 4.1.4 Treatment

During the acute phase the use of NSAIDs or a subacromial injection may be necessary. This followed by physical therapy for rotator cuff strengthening and scapular stabilization exercises. Once the athlete has completed the acute phase of physical therapy (PT), he or she transitions into the maintenance phase. Surgical intervention is rarely indicated for impingement syndrome. Some surgical procedures that are used to treat this syndrome include acromioplasty and arthroscopic repair.

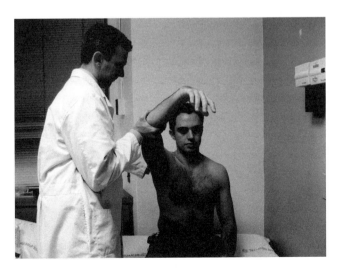

**Fig. 5.2** Neer impingement test

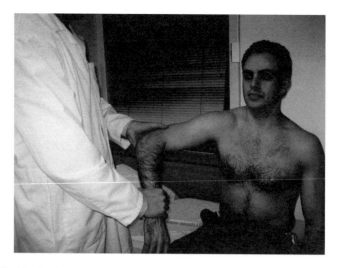

**Fig. 5.3** Hawkins impingement test

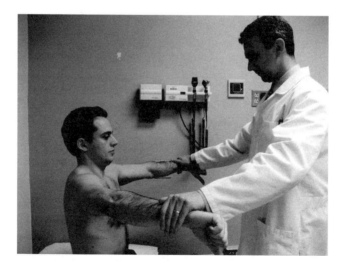

**Fig. 5.4** Empty can test

### 4.1.5 Return to Play

Return to play depends on the severity of the injury and ranges from 4 weeks to 3 months. The athlete may also have to modify his or her body mechanics when playing the sport to prevent recurrent injury.

## *4.2   Shoulder Instability*

Shoulder instability is the pathological tendency of a joint to dislocate causing pain and functional impairment. Instability can be classified as traumatic or atraumatic. Patients with traumatic unidirectional instability with a Bankart lesion (TUBS) usually require surgical intervention. Patients with no history of trauma (atraumatic type) with multidirectional and bilateral instability (AMBRI) are usually treated with physical therapy or surgically with inferior capsular repair. Atraumatic causes include repetitive overuse injury, Marfan's syndrome, and Ehlers-Danlos syndrome. The sport that usually leads to chronic instability due to repetitive overuse is swimming.

Shoulder laxity is a term which has been used interchangeably with instability, but these two terms have to different definitions. Instability refers to a pathological process, whereas laxity refers to the normal, painless freedom of movement around a joint.

### 4.2.1   Clinical Presentation

Athletes with shoulder instability usually present complaining of a feeling that the shoulder is "loose" or about to "pop out." This sense of instability may or may not be accompanied with pain. These patients may also report a prior history of dislocation.

### 4.2.2   Diagnosis

The diagnosis of instability is made clinically. Inspection of the upper extremities may show side-to-side asymmetry. Range of motion testing may reveal hypermobile joints bilaterally in the case of those with multidirectional instability. Specific orthopedic maneuvers are also useful in discerning the type of instability the athlete may have.

- Apprehension test: This test is performed with the patient in the seated or supine position. The shoulder is abducted to 90 degrees with the elbow flexed to 90 degrees (Fig. 5.5A). Once in this position an external rotation force is provided by the examiner. Pain or a sense of impending dislocation is a positive sign for anterior instability.
- Relocation test: This test is performed after the a positive apprehension test is noted. The patient is placed in the same position as above, but a posterior force is placed on the anterior shoulder region (Fig. 5.5B). If the patient allows an increase in external rotation this is a positive test for anterior instability.
- Sulcus sign: This test is performed with the patient in the seated or standing position. The arm is distracted in the inferior direction. If a gap is noted on one side it may indicate inferior instability.

- Jerk test: The shoulder is forward flexed to 90 degrees and the elbow flexed to 90 degrees. A posterior force is placed on the elbow. If the patient reports a sense of dislocation this is a positive test for posterior instability (Fig. 5.6).
- Load-shift test: The patient is seated when the examiner grabs the proximal arm and applies a load through the humeral head. The examiner then places an anterior and posterior force to the shoulder. If the examiner notes excessive movement in comparison to the unaffected shoulder this may indicate anterior, posterior, or multidirectional instability.

Radiological studies may include the use of an MRI to evaluate the soft tissue structures. An MRI is most useful in those with traumatic unidirectional instability in order to asses the presence of a Bankart lesion, which is a tear of the labrum, or Hill-Sachs lesion, which is damage to the cartilaginous surface of the humeral head.

### 4.2.3 Treatment

TUBS injuries usually require surgery but conservative treatment can be attempted prior to considering surgery. Conservative treatment consists of a brief period of sling immobilization for approximately 3 weeks and physical therapy. Therapy

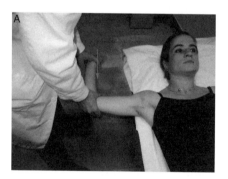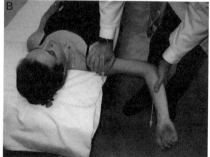

**Fig. 5.5** **A** Apprehension test **B** Relocation test

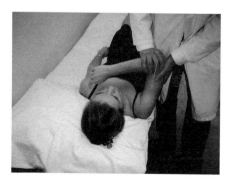

**Fig. 5.6** Jerk test

involves ROM exercises and strengthening of the shoulder girdle muscles. Surgery is considered if therapy fails and involves arthroscopic or open repair.

AMBRI (multidirectional instability) injuries usually respond to physical therapy, which consists of strengthening exercises of the shoulder stabilizers. Stretching exercises of the muscles around the shoulder joint should be avoided. If conservative treatment fails, surgery can be attempted, which usually involves an inferior capsular shift.

### 4.2.4   Return to Play

Patients who have been managed conservatively can return to play once they are pain free and have regained nearly symmetrical ROM and strength in the affected arm. Athletes that have undergone surgery require approximately 6 months prior to returning to their sport. Throwing athletes may require up to 12 months to complete the rehabilitation process prior to returning to play.

## 4.3   Bicipital Tendonitis

Biceps tendonitis is an inflammation of the long head tendon of the biceps. This disorder can result from impingement as it passes through the humeral bicipital groove and inserts on the superior aspect of the labrum of the glenohumeral joint or as an isolated inflammatory injury. Bicipital tendonitis can also be a secondary injury as a result of compensation to other disorders such as labral tears, intra-articular pathology and rotator cuff pathology. Bicipital tendonitis is more common in overhead athletes such as baseball pitchers, swimmers, and tennis player and can be the result of overuse syndrome of the shoulder, which is also common in gymnasts and rowing/kayaking athletes. Trauma may cause direct injury to the tendon as the arm is moved into excessive abduction and external rotation.

### 4.3.1   Clinical Presentation

Athletes usually complain of pain with overhead activity or lifting heavy objects and localize the pain to the anterior shoulder. The patient typically describes the pain as achy in quality. The pain is exacerbated by lifting or elevated pushing or pulling and may improve with rest. Most patients have not sustained an acute traumatic injury, although partial traumatic ruptures have occurred.

### 4.3.2   Diagnosis

Physical exam reveals local tenderness over the bicipital groove and pain with flexion of the elbow against resistance. If the diagnosis is not apparent, other physical exam maneuvers can be used to make the diagnosis such as the Speed test and Yergason test.

### 4.3.3 Special Tests

- *Speed test:* Patient elevates the arm to 90 degrees with the elbow extended and palm upward and having the patient attempt forward flexion of the arm against resistance (Fig. 5.7). Anterior shoulder pain (pain in the bicipital groove) is a positive test.
- *Yergason test:* Patients elbow is flexed to 90 degrees and the arm is against the thorax. The patient is asked to supinate the forearm against resistance (see Fig. 5.4). A positive test is pain and tenderness over the bicipital groove.

Diagnostic studies such as x-rays and MRIs are helpful and should be considered after unsuccessful rehabilitation or when rotator cuff injury is suspected.

### 4.3.4 Treatment

Initial treatment consists of NSAIDs, which can be used for 3–4 weeks to reduce inflammation and pain in addition to rest and the application of ice to the affected area. Patients should also be educated to avoid painful movements such as reaching and lifting. Physical therapy can be performed with the goal of achieving and maintaining full and painless ROM as well as increasing strength and endurance.

### 4.3.5 Return to Play

The athlete can return to play in approximately 3 weeks and/or once pain has resolved completely.

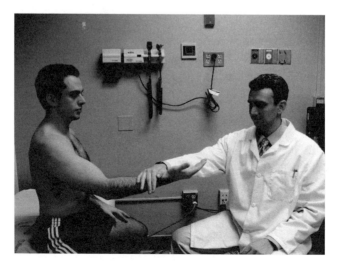

**Fig. 5.7** Speed test

## 4.4   Labral Tears

The labrum is located on the periphery of the glenoid fossa and is a fibrocartilaginous structure that serves to deepen the glenoid. Tendons of the rotator cuff muscles and the biceps insert on the labrum; therefore, any instability or tear of the labrum can be accompanied by biceps tendon or rotator cuff pathology.

The SLAP (Superior Labral Anterior to Posterior) and other glenoid labral tears are common in throwing athletes and athletes involved in repetitive overhead sports such as baseball, tennis, or volleyball. Labral tears can also result from trauma such as a fall on an outstretched arm or direct impact on the shoulder.

### 4.4.1   Clinical Presentation

The athlete presents with a painful shoulder that pops or clicks with motion. The patient may also complain of weakness in the affected arm and a grinding sound or sensation with movement of the shoulder.

### 4.4.2   Diagnosis

Physical exam reveals tenderness to deep palpation over the anterior glenohumeral joint and signs of laxity or instability. Patients often have a positive "clunk" test. If the diagnosis is not apparent by the general physical exam, special tests such as the clunk test can be performed.

### 4.4.3   Special Tests

- *Clunk test:* Patient is supine and patient's arm is rotated and loaded (force applied) from extension through to forward flexion. A "clunk" sound or clicking sensation can indicate a labral tear.
- *O'Brien's test:* Patient's shoulder is adducted and internally rotated. An inferiorly directed force is applied (Fig. 5.8). Then the shoulder is externally rotated and an inferiorly directed force is applied again. If pain is reproduced with resisted force when the shoulder is internally rotated (thumb facing down) but *not* when the shoulder is externally rotated (thumb facing up), it is a positive O'Brien's test.

Diagnostic studies such x-rays may be helpful to rule out other pathology and can reveal if loose bodies are present. MRI may be useful to view the torn labrum.

### 4.4.4   Types of SLAP Injuries

- *Type 1:* Attachment of labrum to the glenoid is intact but there is evidence of fraying and degeneration

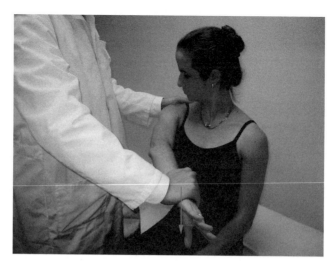

**Fig. 5.8** O'Brien's test

- *Type 2:* Detachment of superior labrum and long-head tendon of the biceps from the glenoid rim
- *Type 3:* Meniscoid superior labrum is torn away and displaced into the joint, but long-head tendon and its labral rim attachment are intact
- *Type 4:* Tear of the superior labrum extends into the long-head tendon, part of which is displaced into the joint along with the superior labrum

### 4.4.5 Treatment

Athletes are treated with rest and NSAIDs as well as physical therapy that focuses on ROM exercises and strengthening exercises of the shoulder girdle muscles. If conservative treatment does not work, then arthroscopic or open surgical repair may be indicated. More specifically, Types 2 and 4 SLAP injuries cause shoulder instability. Arthroscopic reattachment of the labrum to the glenoid is the surgery of choice, whereas Type 1 and 3 SLAP injuries do not cause instability and can be treated with arthroscopic débridement.

### 4.4.6 Return to Play

Athletes may return to play once they are pain free and ROM has been restored. After surgery patients require approximately 2–3 months of rest followed by therapy with focus on ROM and strengthening exercises.

# References

1. Beim GM (2000) Acromioclavicular joint injuries. J Athl Train 35(3):26–267
2. Cox JS (1981) The fate of the acromioclavicular joint in athletic injuries. Am J Sports Med 9(1):50–53
3. DePalma AF (1983) Surgery of the shoulder 3rd edn. Lippincott, Philadelphia
4. Durham BA (1995) Bicipital tendinitis. In: Nicholis JA, Hershman EB (eds) The Upper extremity in sports medicine, 2nd ed. Mosby, St. Louis, 303–306
5. Ernberg LA, Potter HG (2003) Radiographic evaluation of the acromioclavicular and the sternoclavicular joints. Clin Sports Med 22:255–275
6. Fongemie AE, Buss DD, Rolnick SJ (1998) Management of shoulder impingement syndrome and rotator cuff tears. Am Fam Phys 57(4):667–674
7. Friedman RJ, Blocker ER, Morrow DL (1995) Glenohumeral instability. J South Orthop Assoc 4:182–199
8. Gross J, Fetto J, Rosen E (2002) Musculoskeletal examination, 2nd edn. Blackwell Science, Cambridge, MA, 189–191
9. Hawkins RJ, Kennedy JC (1980) Impingement syndrome in athletes. Am J Sports Med 8:151–157
10. Hawkins RJ, Montadi NG (1991) Controversy in anterior shoulder instability. Clin Orthop 272:152–161
11. Iannotti JP, Williams GR (1999) Disorders of the shoulder: diagnosis and management. Lippincott Williams &d Wilkins, Philadelphia
12. Kovacic J, Bergfeld J (2005) Return to play issues in upper extremity injuries. Clin J Sports Med 15(6):448–452
13. Mahaffey BL, Smith PA (1999) Shoulder instability in young athletes. Am Fam Phys 15(10)
14. Murrell GA, Warren RF (1995) The surgical treatment of posterior shoulder instability. Clin Sports Med 14;903–915
15. Murtagh J (1991) Bicipital tendonitis. Aust Fam Phys 20(6):817
16. Neer CS (1983) Impingement lesions. Clin Orthop 173:70–77
17. Park MC, Blaine TA, Levine WN (2002) Shoulder dislocation in young athletes. Phys Sports Med 30(12)
18. Quillen DM, Wuchner M, Hatch RL (2004) Acute shoulder injuries. Am Fam Phys 70: 1947–1954
19. Richards DB (1999) Injuries to the glenoid labrum: a diagnostic and treatment challenge. Phys Sports Med 27(6):41–48
20. Robinson G, Ho Y, Finlay K, Friedman L, Harish S (2006) Normal anatomy and common labral lesions at MR arthrography of the shoulder. Clin Radiol 61(10):805–821
21. Rockwood Jr CA, Williams G, Young C (1996) Injuries to the acromioclavicular joint. In: Rockwood CA Jr. Green D, Bucholz R (eds) Fractures in adults. Lippincott-Raven, Philadelphia, 1341–414
22. Woodward TW, Best TM (2000) The painful shoulder: Part I. Clinical evaluation. Am Fam Phys 61(10):3291–3300

# Chapter 6
# Elbow and Forearm Injuries

Victor Ibrahim and Elise Weiss

## 1 Anatomy of the Elbow

### 1.1 Bones

The elbow is a synovial hinge joint formed by three articulations that arise from the juxtaposition of the humerus, ulna, and radius. The pool-shaped trochlea of the humerus articulates with the ulna to form the humeroulnar joint. The spheroidal capitellum articulates with the concave radial head to form the humeroradial joint. The third joint, radioulnar, is divided into superior and inferior portions. The elbow joint is surrounded by a fibrous capsule, which attaches to the articular margins of the joint and blends into fibers of the elbow's two primary collateral ligaments: medial and lateral.

### 1.2 Nerves

Three important nerves innervate the elbow joint: the median, radial, and ulnar. The ulnar nerve passes from posterior to anterior compartments through a dense sheet of fibrous tissue and continues along the posterior aspect of the medial condyle. It then passes through the cubital tunnel and provides motor innervation to the flexor carpi ulnaris. The median nerve crosses the elbow lateral the ulnar nerve. It dives through the intermuscular system and provides innervation to the anterior elbow and eventually the pronator teres. The radial nerve travels laterally along the spiral groove of the humerus to the lateral epicondyle after which it divides into deep and superficial branches. It eventually provides motor innervation to the wrist extensors and abductor pollicis longus.

### 1.3 Muscles

Several muscles pass through the elbow joint that allow for flexion, extension of the elbow, and pronation and supination of the forearm. Although a weak flexor of the elbow, the pronator teres is a strong pronator of the forearm and is often injured by pitchers. This muscle has two heads that originate from the ulna and medial epicondyle. It is between these heads that median nerves passes through the elbow. Another muscle that passes through the elbow joint is the flexor carpi radialis, which also originates from the medial epicondyle and plays an important role in wrist flexion. The primary muscle of the posterior segment of the elbow is the triceps, which plays a fundamental role in extension. The medial and lateral head of the triceps originate from the scapula and the posterior surface of the humerus and attach at the proximal end of the olecranon and fascia of the forearm. The biceps and brachioradialis are found anteriorly and function as the primary flexors of the elbow. When the forearm is pronated, however, the biceps actually aids in supination. The two heads of the biceps originate from the coracoid process and supraglenoid tubercle and insert into the radius and fascia of the forearm. The brachioradialis originates from the supracondylar ridge of the humerus and inserts into the lateral distal end of the radius. Approximately 95% of the anterior elbow is covered by the brachialis, which is a flexor of the forearm. It originates from the distal anterior half of the humerus and inserts into the coracoid process and tuberosity of the ulna. An important muscle that is involved in elbow pathology is the extensor carpi ulnaris, an important extensor of the wrist. The muscle has two heads, which originate from the ulna and radius and insert into the fifth metacarpal.

## 1.4 Biomechanics

The primary function of the elbow is to stabilize and position the hand. This function is achieved by the coordination of bones, joints, ligaments, and muscles. The four basic movements of the elbow are controlled by different muscle groups. Elbow flexion is controlled by the biceps, brachialis, and brachioradialis. Despite having a smallest cross-sectional area, the brachioradialis plays the most significant role in flexion because of its mechanical advantage. Extension of the elbow is achieved primarily by the triceps, with a small amount of help from the anconeus muscle. Pronation of the elbow is controlled by the pronator quadratus, pronator teres, and flexor carpi radialis. The supinators of the elbow include the supinator and biceps brachii muscles. The medial and lateral epicondyles of the humerus are home two the basic wrist flexors and extensors, respectively.

The average ROM in the elbow is 0–145 degrees; however, studies suggest that only 30–145 degrees are needed for most activities of daily living. Different joints play unique roles in elbow movement. The humeroulnar joint's primary function is flexion, extension, and stability, whereas the primary function of the humeroradial joint allows for flexion, extension, and axial rotation. Further stability is gained from the medial and lateral collateral ligaments. Although both of these ligaments insert on the medial border of the ulna, the thicker anterior band is the most important valgus stabilizer. The normal ROM for forearm supination is 90 degrees, whereas it is only 80 degrees for pronation.

## 2  Elbow Injuries

### 2.1  Lateral Epicondylitis

Commonly referred to as tennis elbow (frequency includes 75% of club tennis players), lateral epicondylitis is the most common overuse injury of the elbow. It is an injury to the extensor tendons (i.e., extensor carpi radialis) that arises from repetitive microtrauma and overload.

#### 2.1.1  Presentation

Patients commonly complain of worsening aching pain over the lateral elbow, which is worse with movement and alleviated by rest. In more chronic cases, however, the pain may be persistent and associated with forearm weakness.

#### 2.1.2  Diagnosis

Diagnosis is based primarily on physical exam and history. Pain is elicited on palpation of the lateral epicondyle, and is aggravated by wrist extension and radial deviation. In Cozen's test (Fig. 6.1) the patient extends the wrist against resistance that is provided by the examiner at the same time as the examiner palpates the lateral epicondyle. In lateral epicondylitis, this will be very painful. In more severe cases, decreased grip strength can be noted. MRI or ultrasound can be used for diagnosis, but is usually reserved for patients who fail conservative therapy.

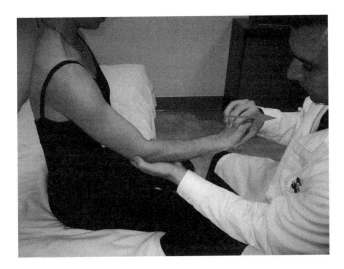

**Fig. 6.1** Cozen's test

### 2.1.3  Treatment

Initial treatment includes NSAIDs, RICE (rest, ice, compress, elevate), and activity modification. Long-term treatment should focus on ROM exercises. Although bracing is a common treatment, continuous immobilization can actually be harmful, as studies have suggested that the tendons need stress to heal. There is evidence that steroid injection provides a short-term benefit at 4 weeks versus NSAIDs alone. Surgery is rarely needed and is reserved for those with significant decrease in arm strength. Surgery is only capable of restoring 90% of the tensile strength.

In addition, tennis players should be sure to check the grip size on their racquet. Inappropriate grip size, higher string tensions in the racquet, and poor stroke mechanics can all contribute to lateral epicondylitis. A tennis player who develops lateral epicondylitis should have all of these factors evaluated and addressed.

### 2.1.4  Return to Play

Play can be resumed when an athlete has full strength and is able to complete all necessary movements without pain. A brace may be used temporarily, but athletes must continue to participate in a therapy program while recovering.

## 2.2  *Medial Epicondylitis*

Commonly referred to as golfer's elbow, medial epicondylitis is an injury to the common flexor tendons (i.e., flexor carpi radialis). Compared with lateral epicondylitis, it is seen <10% of the time, and results from repetitive microtrauma from valgus stress on the medial epicondyle.

### 2.2.1  Presentation

Athletes typically present with pain and tenderness over the medial elbow. In more chronic cases, weakness can be reported the forearm and wrist.

### 2.2.2  Diagnosis

Diagnosis is based primarily on physical exam and history. Pain on palpation of the medial epicondyle is often seen, and in 20% of cases ulnar nerve symptoms (i.e., numbness, weakness) can be noted on the exam. Passive extension of the elbow and wrist and supination of the elbow can also elicit symptoms and is suggestive of a positive diagnosis. Resisted wrist flexion with palpation of the medial epicondyle also may reproduce symptoms (Fig. 6.2). Imaging studies are often unnecessary, but may show calcification adjacent to the medial epicondyle in 20% of affected patients.

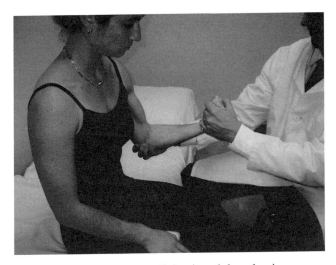

**Fig. 6.2** Resisted wrist flexion with medial epicondyle palpation

### 2.2.3 Treatment

Initial treatment includes NSAIDs, RICE, and activity modification.

Physical therapy emphasizing ROM and strengthening are important strategies. Steroid injection shows effective short-term relief, but no evidence suggests that there is long-term benefit. Counterforce bracing and taping can be useful when return to play is a pressing priority. Surgery is reserved for cases that fail conservative treatment, but have a longer recovery time (4–6 months).

Golfers should have their stroke evaluated. Poor stroke biomechanics can contribute to medial epicondylitis. Tennis players should have their stroke evaluated. Excessive topspin in tennis and other racquet sports may lead to medial epicondylitis.

### 2.2.4 Return to Play

Athletes may ideally return to play when pain has resolved with activity. Since most athletes are unwilling to wait, bracing and activity modification are often used to reduce the amount of off-time.

## 2.3 Olecranon Bursitis (Draftsman's Elbow)

Olecranon bursitis is an inflammation of the bursa overlying the olecranon process at the proximal aspect of the ulna. The bursa is located between the ulna and the skin at the posterior tip of the elbow. Bursal inflammation occurs by a variety of mechanisms, including acute or repetitive trauma. Less commonly, the inflammation may be due to infection.

### 2.3.1  Clinical Presentation

Patients complain of pain and focal swelling at the posterior elbow. Pain tends to be exacerbated with pressure on the area. Onset can be chronic or acute, but when acute a history of trauma is usually noted.

### 2.3.2  Diagnosis

The most classic physical finding is swelling over the olecranon process. If the area is red or warm, infection should be considered. Elbow ROM is usually normal because the bursa is extra-articular, but occasionally movement may be limited by pain. Radiographs of the elbow should be performed to assess for possible olecranon fracture if significant trauma occurred or an avulsed osteophyte is suspected. Bursal aspiration is the standard to differentiate septic and aseptic olecranon bursitis. Given the risk associated with infection, every patient with acute bursitis must undergo aspiration, as physical exam can not alone distinguish septic from aseptic bursitis. Definitive diagnosis occurs with laboratory evaluation of cell count, gram stain, and crystal analysis.

### 2.3.3  Treatment

In the absence of infection, most patients respond very well to a series of one to two aspirations (with or without corticosteroid injection) combined with ice and rest. Although compression of the area is indicated, application of excessive pressure should be avoided.

### 2.3.4  Return to Play

The athlete is able to return to play without restriction when symptoms and physical examination findings resolve. A good test for return is participation in sport-specific practice drills. If there is no recurrence of symptoms or findings on physical exam the athlete is considered clear for activity.

## 2.4  Little League Elbow

Commonly a result of the valgus stress during repetitive throwing movements, little league elbow is an injury to the supporting structures of the medical elbow. This microtrauma results in three classic findings: (1) medial epicondylitis, (2) traction apophysitis, and (3) delayed or accelerated growth of the medial epicondyle. Delayed diagnosis and treatment can lead to growth plate disruption, leading to permanent deformity.

### 2.4.1 Presentation

Although athletes most often present with medial elbow pain, lateral and posterior pain can be provoked with palpation. Pain is most commonly elicited during the cocking and/or accelerating phase of throwing. Importantly, pain during the deceleration phase is more suggestive of a posterior elbow injury.

### 2.4.2 Diagnosis

History and physical are the primary tools of diagnosis. Radiographic studies can be helpful when the diagnosis is unclear, or other pathology such as fracture is suspected.

### 2.4.3 Treatment

Treatment is determined by the chronicity of disease. In the acute phase, RICE and physical therapy are important. In more severe and chronic conditions, casting or surgery may be required. Oral NSAIDs may be used for pain control, but no evidence suggests that steroid injection is helpful.

### 2.4.4 Return to Play

Most athletes can return to play within 4–6 weeks or after the completion of a rehabilitation program. Gradual return to throwing with proper technique should be emphasized.

## 2.5 Pronator Syndrome

The most common site of median nerve forearm entrapment is under the hypertrophied head of the pronator muscle. Other areas include the lacertus fibrosus at the elbow or under the flexor digitorum superficialis.

### 2.5.1 Clinical Presentation

Patients often complain of pain or paresthesias in the median nerve distribution with prominent complaints in the anterior proximal forearm. A patient may note that throwing or swinging a racquet aggravates the pain.

### 2.5.2 Diagnosis

Patients often present with a hypertrophied pronator muscle. Median nerve symptoms with negative Tinel and Phalen tests at the wrist should raise suspicion of pronator syndrome. A Tinel sign over the proximal forearm (pronator muscle) and increased pain with resisted pronation are also consistent with this diagnosis. Athletes with pronator syndrome have difficulty touching the tips of the first and second fingers to make a circle (the OK sign). This is consistent with weakness in the median nerve distribution. Specifically, motor loss is noted in decreased ability to pronate and flex the wrist as well as partial loss of finger flexion and loss of thumb opposition. A key distinguishing feature between pronator syndrome and carpal tunnel syndrome is the decreased sensation over the thenar eminence that is unique to pronator syndrome. This is because the sensory branch of the median nerve (palmar cutaneous branch) innervating the thenar eminence does not pass through the tunnel. As probably suspected, electrodiagnostic testing can provide evidence for the diagnosis of pronator syndrome.

### 2.5.3   Treatment

Treatment of pronator syndrome involves rest, modification of daily activities, NSAIDS and an elbow splint. After pain subsides the athlete can begin simple hand exercises (ball squeeze). This can progress to light wrist flexion and extension and then pronation and supination exercises. If this treatment fails for 4–6 weeks, surgical exploration can be considered and an anatomical exploration for nerve compression can be sought.

### 2.5.4   Return to Play

Return to play is usually appropriate when pain is resolved and the cause for compression is addressed through either biomechanical or anatomical changes. Strength should be 100% of the unaffected side at the time of return to activity.

## 2.6   Anterior Interosseous Nerve Syndrome (Kiloh Nevin Syndrome)

Anterior interosseous syndrome involves the median nerve as it divides approximately 5 cm below the lateral epicondyle of the elbow. The anterior interosseous nerve innervates the flexor pollicis longus, the radial half of the flexor digitorum profundus, and the pronator quadratus.

### 2.6.1   Clinical Presentation

Symptoms may include vague pain in the proximal forearm and weakness in the nerve's distribution. The patient usually describes acute onset of weakness in the thumb and index finger. The patient may also note a loss of coordination of the fingers.

## 2.6.2 Diagnosis

Since the anterior interosseous nerve is a purely motor nerve, clinical weakness in its distribution is diagnostic. Patients are classically unable to form the OK sign with the thumb and second digit. The thumb index finger pinch is abnormal with no flexion of the distal interphalangeal joint (DIP), of the index finger and hyperextension of the interphalageal joint (IP) joint of the thumb. There may also be a compensatory increase in flexion of the proximal intraphalangeal joint (PIP) joint of the finger. This pinch is characteristic of anterior interosseous syndrome. Electrodiagnostic studies can provide further evidence to confirm the clinically suspected diagnosis.

## 2.6.3 Treatment

Conservative treatment is the initial intervention of choice. This includes relative rest, ice and pain control. If no improvement is seen in 6–8 weeks, surgical exploration is indicated.

## 2.6.4 Return to Play

Return to play is usually appropriate when pain is resolved and the cause for compression is resolved either through biomechanical or anatomical changes. Strength should be 100% of the unaffected side at the time of return to activity.

## 2.7 Fractures and Dislocation

Elbow dislocation is the second most common dislocation in adults (second to shoulder) and the most common in children. Elbow dislocations are considered simple or complex. Simple dislocations involve posterior (90% of cases) or anterior translocation. Complex dislocations involve fracture and nerve damage. A classic complex dislocation, the Essex-Lopresti fracture-dislocation, involves a comminuted radial head fracture and a distal radioulnar joint dislocation. Patients often report a history of high-velocity impact and falling on an outstretched hand (FOOSH) as the primary mode of injury. Elbow fractures fall into three basic categories: (1) fractures of the proximal ulna, (2) fractures of the proximal radius, and (3) fractures of the distal humerus.

## 2.7.1 Presentation

Severe pain in the elbow after a FOOSH injury is common. Numbness (i.e., medial, radial, and ulnar nerve damage) and weakness can be seen in more severe cases.

## 2.7.2 Diagnosis

Although physical and history are sufficient to diagnose dislocation, plain radiographic studies are important for treatment considerations. When fracture is suspected, anteroposterior (AP) view in full extension and lateral view in 90-degree flexion should be obtained. Smaller fracture may not be visible on x-ray initially, but may become more evident 3 weeks postinjury. In children, oblique views may be more helpful when fractures are not evident and the fat pad is displaced. Supracondylar fractures, which are most common in children, can be often confused with dislocation. More complex fractures may require CT imaging to visualize bony fragments. Dislocation-fracture injuries can be classified into four types based on frequency and character (see Table 6.1).

## 2.7.3 Treatment

For simple dislocation, reduction on the field or in the office is the primary treatment. Pre- and postreduction films are important to rule out fracture and ensure proper alignment. Physical therapy emphasizing ROM is important after the immediate acute phase. Splinting for >3 weeks may be adverse. For most nondisplaced elbow fractures, immobilization is the primary treatment. Displaced fractures require surgical intervention (i.e., ORIF). Minimally or nondisplaced radial head fractures require fluid aspiration, 1–2 splinting and then early mobilization. Type III or displaced fractures require surgical intervention.

## 2.7.4 Return to Play

After a simple dislocation, most athletes can return to play after 3–6 weeks. Compliance with a rehabilitation program is important to emphasize. Previous elbow dislocation does not predispose athletes to repeat injury. Athletes with nerve injury

**Table 6.1** Bado classification of monteggia fracture-dislocation

| Type | Description | Frequency, %* |
|---|---|---|
| I | Fracture of the middle or proximal third of the ulna and anterior dislocation of the radial head | 65 |
| II | Fracture of the middle or proximal third of the ulna and posterior dislocation of the radial head | 18 |
| III | Ulnar fracture distal to the coronoid process with lateral radial head dislocation | 16 |
| IV | Fracture of the proximal or middle third of the ulna with an anterior dislocation of the radial head and fracture of the proximal third of the radius | 1 |

*Bado Classification of Monteggia Fracture-Dislocation (adapted from Resnick, 2002).
Radial head fractures are classified based on Mason's classification. Type I is non-displaced, Type II is displaced, and Type III is comminuted fracture.

(up to 15%) should be monitored regularly. Complex dislocation and elbow fractures require more extensive rehabilitation, valgus bracing and return to play is often recommended 6 months postinjury. Again, emphasis is placed on range motion during therapy and bracing to avoid valgus stress on the elbow during rigorous play.

## 2.8 Cubital Tunnel Syndrome

Also referred to as ulnar nerve entrapment, cubital tunnel syndrome is the second most common nerve compression disorder. (The first is carpal tunnel.) The pathway of the ulnar nerve predisposes it to compressive, traction, and friction forces. The cubital tunnel is found deep to the arcuate, which connects the ulnar and humeral heads of the flexor carpi ulnaris (FCU) muscle. Repeat elbow flexion can cause irritation of the ulnar nerve through this tunnel and lead to nerve irritation and dysfunction.

### 2.8.1 Presentation

Athletes present with complaints of numbness and tingling in the elbow and lateral hand, especially the fifth digit. The quality and quantity of discomfort can vary greatly and muscle weakness can be noted in more chronic or severe cases.

### 2.8.2 Diagnosis

History and physical are the primary tools of diagnosis. A positive elbow flexion test is the most classic and common finding. In this test, the patient will complain of discomfort with supination of the forearm, extension of the wrist and flexion of the elbow past 90 degrees after 3 or more minutes (or sometimes sooner). Palpation of the ulnar nerve as it passes through the elbow (in the area commonly referred to as "the funny bone") can also reproduce symptoms (Fig. 6.3). A thorough neurological and muscular examination should be done to rule out other pathologies. In the setting of trauma, imaging including ultrasound, plain films, and MRI should be considered. One study suggests that radiographic abnormalities can be seen in as many as 29% of patients. Vague physical exams may warrant further evaluation with EMG.

### 2.8.3 Treatment

Treatment varies depending on etiology. Physical therapy, including strengthening and stretching along with oral NSAIDs, should be considered. Splinting the elbow in extension at night to avoid further injury may also be helpful. Steroid injections are often avoided due to nerve damage complications. Surgery should be considered when conservative therapy fails.

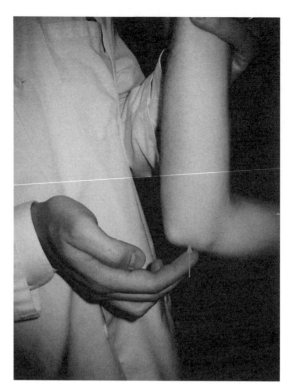

**Fig. 6.3** Ulnar nerve palpation at the elbow

### 2.8.4  Return to Play

Recovery and return to play vary depending on therapy and response time. When athletes are asymptomatic with full ROM, they may resume play with continued therapy and movement modification.

## 2.9  Triceps Tendinitis

Most commonly seen in weight lifters, triceps tendinitis is inflammation and degeneration of the triceps tendon at its insertion into the olecranon.

### 2.9.1  Presentation

Athletes present with posterior elbow pain, which is worse with elbow extension, and exacerbated by resistance. Chronic cases can present with decreased ROM and a palpable depression along the olecranon process.

### 2.9.2 Diagnosis

History and physical are the primary tools of diagnosis. If triceps tendon rupture is suspected, imaging including MRI should be considered. Plain films may show calcification along the tendon line.

### 2.9.3 Treatment

The primary treatment is RICE and NSAIDs. Physical therapy emphasizing triceps strengthening is important in long-term treatment. Steroid injection is avoided due to the risk of tendon rupture.

### 2.9.4 Return to Play

Return to play is acceptable when symptoms are tolerable, activity modification is addressed and strength is at least 90% of baseline.

## 2.10 Triceps Rupture

Avulsion of the triceps tendon is a rare event that most often is the result of a deceleration stress superimposed on a contracted triceps muscle. Some case reports suggest a higher prevalence among athletes who abuse anabolic steroids. Rupture of the tendon can occur at three places: the tendon attachment to bone, the musculotendinous junction, or in the muscle body itself.

### 2.10.1 Presentation

Athletes most commonly present with posterior elbow pain and weakness. The classic presentation is weakness of elbow extension and a palpable gap in the muscle body. In the setting of acute trauma, ecchymosis or localized tenderness can be appreciated.

### 2.10.2 Diagnosis

History and physical are the primary tools of diagnosis. MRI studies should be considered when the diagnosis is unclear, but should be use with caution as studies suggest a false-negative prevalence.

### 2.10.3   Treatment

Nonsurgical treatment including physical therapy, RICE, and NSAIDs is most often utilized. The role of surgical intervention remains an area of discussion in most cases.

### 2.10.4   Return to Play

Athletes may return to play when full ROM and symptoms have resolved.

## 2.11   Elbow Hyperextension Injury

Elbow hyperextension injury is often the result of a high-velocity impact, resulting in overextension of the elbow joint. Damage to ligaments and flexor tendons (i.e., biceps) can be observed.

### 2.11.1   Presentation

Athletes often present with posterior elbow pain and pain with palpation of the of the biceps tendon.

### 2.11.2   Diagnosis

History and physical are the primary tools of diagnosis. If fracture or ligament rupture is suspected, MRI may be warranted for further evaluation.

### 2.11.3   Treatment

Initial treatment in the acute phase includes RICE and NSAIDs. Bracing using tape or hyperextension braces should be considered.

### 2.11.4   Return to Play

Athletes may return to play when symptoms resolve and may require taping and bracing during activity.

## 2.12   Distal Biceps Tendon Rupture

Rupture of the proximal biceps tendon comprises 90–97% of all biceps ruptures and almost exclusively involves the long head. Distal biceps tendon ruptures account for the remainder. Predisposition to this rare rupture occurs with degeneration of the tendon. When forceful extension is applied to a flexed elbow this already weakened structure can rupture.

### 2.12.1 Clinical Presentation

Distal biceps tendon rupture is characterized by sudden pain over the anterior aspect of the elbow after a forceful effort against resistance. Usually the patient will hear a snap and have pain when the tendon rupture occurs. Swelling and bruising are soon to follow and a visible or palpable mass may develop in the upper arm.

### 2.12.2 Diagnosis

History is often suggestive of diagnosis. Elbow and shoulder ROM should be evaluated and complete strength testing should be performed. The arm contour is very revealing with regard to diagnosis. The Ludington test (or position), in which the hands are clasped behind the head and the biceps muscle is flexed, is often used to evaluate the contour of the arm. Other maneuvers, such as the Speed test and Yergason sign, are used to identify patients who may have partial tears, or who may be predisposed to future rupture. Plain radiographs may reveal hypertrophic spurring or bony irregularities that increase the likelihood of rupture and support a clinical suspicion of this diagnosis. Anteroposterior and axillary films are the most useful views for ruling out fractures in this setting. Although arthrography can be used to further diagnose tendon rupture, increasingly ultrasound and MRI are employed.

### 2.12.3 Treatment

Treatment of biceps tendon rupture is a topic of debate. Generally accepted clinical guidelines advocate anatomical reattachment for young or athletic patients or those who require maximum supination strength. Cosmetic concerns may also prompt a surgical approach. Regardless of indication, intervention must be made quickly before the tendon contracts. Conservative management is considered appropriate for middle-aged or older patients and for those who do not require a high degree of supination strength in daily activities. This approach involves rest, followed closely by ROM and strengthening exercises for the shoulder and elbow. When conservative management is chosen, a significant reduction in power should be expected.

### 2.12.4 Return to Play

It takes months for the tendon to form a strong attachment to the bone, so the recovery phase is long. During recovery, heavy use of the arm, especially for pulling and lifting, should be avoided. A gradual increase in motion and strength training is required. This should progress over many months to full return to sport.

## *2.13   MCL Laxity and Tommy John Surgery*

Named after the famous left-handed pitcher, Tommy John surgery is more formally named medial collateral ligament (MCL) replacement. With the repetitive strain during activities like throwing in baseball, athletes put repetitive stress on the MCL, resulting in eventual laxity.

### 2.13.1   Presentation

Athletes most commonly present with medial elbow pain and swelling. Valgus stress at 25% elbow flexion can help localize the pain.

### 2.13.2   Diagnosis

History and physical along with MRI imaging are needed for definitive diagnosis. Plain films may be initially done to rule out fracture. Arthroscopy can also be used for a definitive diagnosis. A neurological assessment should be done to rule out ulnar nerve injury.

### 2.13.3   Treatment

Conservative management includes relative rest, bracing, and physical therapy to emphasize strengthening, joint stability, and stretching. Surgical intervention should be considered for athletes who fail conservative therapy. A brace to prevent valgus stress should be used in the postoperative period.

### 2.13.4   Return to Play

Most athletes will require a period of 3–6 months after conservative therapy and 9–12 months postsurgery to resume full play.

## References

1. Nirschl RP, Kraushaar BS (1996) Assessment and treatment guidelines for elbow injuries. Phys Sportsmed 24(5):43–60
2. Pappas A (1995) Elbow anatomy and function from upper extremity injuries in the athlete. Churchill Livingstone, London, 303–314

# Chapter 7
# Hand and Wrist Injuries

Elise Weiss

## 1  Anatomy of the Hand and Wrist

### 1.1  Bones

The wrist is formed by articulation of the radius, ulna, and carpal bones, of which there are eight. The radiocarpal joint is formed by the distal radius, scaphoid, and lunate. The ulna does not articulate with the carpal bones. Instead a fibrocartilage triangle sits between the distal ulna and triquetrum. The scaphoid bone links the proximal carpal bones (lunate, triquetrum) and the distal carpal bones (trapezium, trapezoid, capitate, and hamate). The distal row of carpal bones joins to the metacarpal bones to form the carpometacarpal joint. The hand has five metacarpal bones. From proximal to distal there is a base, shaft, and head of the metacarpal. Moving distally are the five metacarpophalangeal joints. This links the phalanges to the metacarpals. MCP joints can flex, extend, abduct, and adduct. Using a combination of these movements, they can move in restricted circumduction. Strong palmar and collateral ligaments support the joints. Additionally, the deep transverse metacarpal ligaments connect the medial four joints to each other and hold the head of the metacarpal bones together. The hand has 14 phalanges. Each digit contains three phalanges and the thumb contains two. More distally there are the simple hinge joints of the phalanges; the proximal and distal interphalangeal joints. Palmar and collateral ligaments support the joints in flexion and extension.

### 1.2  Nerves

All of the nerves that travel to the hand cross the wrist. Three main nerves begin together at the shoulder: the radial nerve, the median nerve, and the ulnar nerve. These nerves carry signals from the brain to the muscles that move the arm, hand, fingers, and thumb. The radial nerve provides sensory innervation to the dorsum of the hand, thumb, index, middle, and part of the ring finger. The median nerve enters the hand through the carpal tunnel and provides motor and sensory innervation to

J.E. Herrera and G. Cooper (eds.), *Essential Sports Medicine*,
doi: 10.1007/978-1-59745-414-8, © Humana Press 2008

much of the hand. Specifically, the median nerve supplies the thenar muscles and the two radial lumbrical muscles. Sensory innervation is provided to the palmar surface of the thumb, index, middle, and part of the ring finger. The ulnar nerve innervates the hypothenar muscles, the ulnar two lumbrical muscles and the interosseous muscles. It also provides sensory innervation to the fifth digit and part of the ring finger.

## 1.3   Muscles

Wrist motion is accomplished primarily by the flexor carpi radialis and ulnaris (major wrist flexors) as well as the extensor carpi radialis and ulnaris (major wrist extensors). Rotators of the wrist include the pronator teres, pronator quadratus, and the supinator.

The superficial forearm contains a large number of muscles that are divided into dorsal and ventral compartments. Dorsally, there are the extensors of the wrist and fingers. They attach to a common extensor origin on the lateral epicondyle of the humerus. Ventrally, the superficial flexors have a common origin on the medial epicondyle of the humerus.

The muscles in the ventral flexor compartment also include extrinsic hand muscles. Their force is transmitted to the hand through long tendons. The deeper flexor digitorum profundus attaches more distally on the fingers than the superficial flexor digitorum superficialis, which means that the FDS tendon has to split to let the FDP pass through it.

The intrinsic muscles of the hand include the lumbricals, interossei, hypothenar, and thenar groups. The lumbricals are muscles that attach to the tendons of the flexor digitorum profundus muscles and the extensor digitorum communalis tendons. They flex the MCP joint and extend the IP joint. The interosseous muscles are located in the intervals between the metacarpal bones. The interossei consist of both dorsal and palmar muscles. The interossei act to abduct (palmar) and adduct (dorsal) the MCP joints of the finger.

Four small muscles of the thumb are found in the thenar side of the hand. These muscles are the abductor pollicis brevis, flexor pollicis brevis, opponens pollicis, and adductor pollicis. The first three of these muscles constitute the thenar eminence. The thenar muscles originate from the flexor retinaculum and carpal bones. The thenar muscles insert onto the base of the thumb or onto the side of the first metacarpal bone. The median nerve innervates the thenar muscles, except the adductor pollicis, which is supplied by the deep branch of the ulnar nerve. In addition to the thenar muscles, there is the abductor pollicis longus, which inserts onto the base of the thumb but originates at the posterior surfaces of the ulna and radius. It acts to abduct the thumb and extend the carpometacarpal joint.

Three small muscles of the little finger are found in the hypothenar side of the hand and are innervated by the ulnar nerve. These muscles are the abductor digiti minimi, flexor digiti minimi, and opponens digiti minimi. The hypothenar muscles originate from the flexor retinaculum and carpal bones. The hypothenar muscles insert onto the base of the fifth metacarpal.

## 1.4  Biomechanics

The radiocarpal joint provides for the majority of wrist flexion, extension, ulnar deviation, and radial deviation. When all motions are taken in combination the wrist can be circumducted. The way that the wrist makes these movements is complex but flexion occurs primarily at the midcarpal joint and extension at the radiocarpal joint. Radial and ulnar collateral ligaments as well as palmar and dorsal radiocarpal ligaments strengthen the joint.

The primary movers of the wrist have dual action. The flexor carpi radialis (FCR) produces wrist flexion and radial deviation, the flexor carpi ulnaris (FCU) produces flexion and ulnar deviation, the extensor carpi radialis (ECR) produces extension and radial deviation, and the extensor carpi ulnaris (ECU) produces extension and ulnar deviation. To produce pure flexion, extension, radial deviation, or ulnar deviation requires activation of the correct two muscles. As an example, the two flexors produce pure flexion because the associated radial and ulnar movements negate one another.

The primary role of the hand is grasping and manipulation. These fine movements are controlled by intrinsic hand muscles. The superficial palmar ventral group includes the thenar and hypothenar eminences, which move the thumb and fifth digit, respectively. The thumb is rotated 90 degrees in relation to the digits so that flexion of the thumb moves it medially across the palm of the hand, abduction moves it anteriorly, extension moves it laterally, and adduction moves it posteriorly. The special movement of opposition is the combined flexion and adduction that brings the palmar surface of the tip of the first digit toward the palmar surface of the tips of any of the other four digits.

The tendon arrangement around the fingers is complex. The flexor digitorum profundus (FDP) tendon pierces the FDS tendon to attach to the base of the distal phalanx and the lumbricals attach to the FDP tendon to the extensor digitorum communis (EDC). The EDC tendon connects to the lumbricals, the dorsal interossei, and all three phalanges and is known as the extensor expansion. This arrangement allows complex movements such as unscrewing a pen top while holding it in the same hand.

## 2  Wrist and Hand Injuries

## 2.1  De Quervain's Tenosynovitis

De Quervain's tenosynovitis is an inflammation of the sheath of the extensor pollicis brevis and abductor pollicis longus tendons due to repetitive or direct trauma to the thumb tendons as they pass over the distal radial styloid. If left untreated, inflammation may convert to fibrosis with a resultant loss in flexibility of the thumb. When this occurs it is known as stenosing tenosynovitis.

### 2.1.1 Clinical Presentation

Common complaints are pain and tenderness on the radial side of the wrist, loss of grip strength, and localized swelling over the radial styloid.

### 2.1.2 Diagnosis

Diagnosis is made largely on history and physical exam. Imaging is not generally necessary except perhaps to rule out other pathology. Physical signs include swelling and tenderness as well as a grating sensation when the thumb is moved. Physical exam assesses the area of tenderness, thumb range of motion and provocative maneuvers. In Finkelstein's test, pain is elicited by passively stretching the thumb tendons over the radial styloid while the thumb is flexed (Fig. 7.1). Diagnosis can be confirmed by an anesthetic block over the radial styloid.

### 2.1.3 Treatment

Noninvasive methods of treatment include application of ice at the radial styloid and the use of a dorsal hood splint or thumb spica splint. The available evidence shows that steroid injection is the most effective treatment, with about 70% of

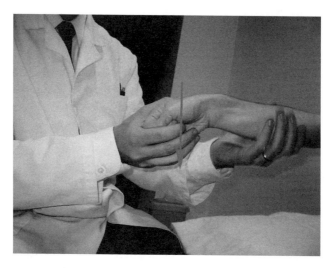

**Fig. 7.1** Finkelstein's test

patients responding to the maximum of two injections. Injections should be spaced at least 6 weeks apart. Surgical intervention is generally not considered until failure of 1 year of conservative management. Physical therapy does not play a prominent role in treatment of De Quervain's tenosynovitis. It does, however, play a role in preventing recurrence. Stretching the extensor and abductor tendons into the palm can be performed in sets of 20 with each stretch being held for 5 seconds.

### 2.1.4 Return to Play

After injection, gripping, grasping, and direct pressure over the styloid should be avoided for 3 days. The wrist should be protected for 3–4 weeks with a thumb spica splint.

## 2.2 Wrist Sprain

Given that human instinct is to use one's hands to break a fall when losing balance, the wrist is at high risk for injury. A wrist sprain occurs as a result of sudden forceful action at the wrist that pushes the natural laxity of supporting ligaments beyond their maximal capacity. It is generally a diagnosis of exclusion. A sprain should be distinguished from a fracture or a strain that involves injury to either muscle or tendon. Wrist sprains are graded according to severity of injury, with grade I being mild and grade III being severe (see following list). Given the risk inherent to certain activities, protective splints in sports such as rollerblading, street hockey, and snowboarding can help prevent many sprained wrists. Other recommendations include not using a pole secured to the wrist while skiing.

### 2.2.1 Grading of Wrist Sprain

- *Grade I:* Mild injury, the ligaments are stretched but not torn
- *Grade II:* Moderate injuries, partial tear of ligaments
- *Grade III:* Severe injury, ligaments are completely torn with resultant joint instability

### 2.2.2 Clinical Presentation

Common complaints when presenting to a physician are pain with movement of the wrist, swelling around the joint, and bruising.

### 2.2.3   Diagnosis

The diagnosis of wrist sprain is made based on history and physical exam. X-ray can rule out fracture.

### 2.2.4   Treatment

Treatment of a wrist sprain in the absence of instability is initially by the RICE method (rest, ice, compress, elevate). The first 24–48 hours are a critical treatment period during which all activities must be avoided. The wrist should gradually be used after this period as tolerated by pain. The principle of the first 48 hours is damage control. Ice should be applied to the wrist for 20 minutes every 3–4 hours. The wrist should be elevated and compressed using an Ace bandage. The bandage should be wrapped from the base of the fingers all the way up to the top of the forearm. This should be done by overlapping the elastic wrap by half the width of the wrap with each time around the forearm. If the fingers become cold, numb, or tingle, the wrap is too tight and should be adjusted. After the initial period of treatment, the patient advances to rehabilitation exercises aimed at restoring function.

### 2.2.5   Return to Play

The amount of rehabilitation and the time needed for recovery depend on the severity of injury and an individual's rate of healing. A mild sprain may take as little as 3–6 weeks to recover while a more severe sprain can take up to 8–12 months. In general, sport can be performed as tolerated after the initial days of healing. If the sport carries increased risk, protective gear is recommended until there is full healing of the injury.

## 2.3   *Navicular (Scaphoid) Fracture*

### 2.3.1   Clinical Presentation

Scaphoid fractures are the most common carpal bone fracture and are typically associated with a fall on an outstretched arm while the wrist is dorsiflexed. If a patient presents early, the key examination finding is tenderness in the anatomical snuffbox. This may be accompanied by swelling and loss of grip strength. A more specific clinical test for acute scaphoid fracture is pain on axial compression of the thumb toward the radius or direct pressure on the scaphoid tuberosity with radial deviation of the wrist. Since pain may improve soon after the fall, a patient may not present to a clinician until late after the injury. This late presentation puts the patient at risk for avascular necrosis. Only one small artery enters the bone, at the end that is closest to the thumb. If the fracture tears the artery, the blood supply is lost and avascular necrosis is the ultimate result.

### 2.3.2 Diagnosis

Tenderness in the anatomical snuff box necessitates a scaphoid fracture being confidently ruled out. Plain x-ray with scaphoid views will usually demonstrate the fracture. A normal x-ray does not exclude the diagnosis of a fracture. In cases in which imaging is negative but clinical suspicion is high, MRI or bone scan can reveal the pathology. If a MRI or bone scan is not available, the wrist should be immobilized for 12 days giving the fracture time to present on x-ray. In patients presenting months after injury, avascular necrosis can be visible on x-ray.

### 2.3.3 Treatment

Most literature suggests that suspicion for a scaphoid fracture warrants immediate placement in a thumb spica splint or cast until radiographic confirmation can be obtained. If a nondisplaced distal fracture is diagnosed, treatment entails a short arm thumb spica cast in slight extension with the thumb IP joint left free. A distal pole fracture should be immobilized for 4–6 weeks, a waist fracture 10–12 weeks, and a proximal pole fracture 12–20 weeks. These are guidelines and as a rule, immobilization should be continued until union is documented on serial radiographs. Following immobilization of a scaphoid fracture, the patient is left with a stiff wrist joint and wasted thenar muscles. Mobilization of the joint should begin immediately after plaster removal. For a fracture displaced >1 mm, presence of altered scapholunate angle or documented nonunion, immediate orthopedic evaluation is warranted as ORIF may be indicated.

### 2.3.4 Return to Play

Nondisplaced fractures that are treated with a short arm thumb spica cast can participate in sport after initial healing is documented. After removal of the spica, the wrist should be protected by a rigid splint for an additional 2 months or until the strength in the affected wrist is at least 80% of uninjured side. Rapid return to sport can be achieved after an open reduction and internal fixation surgery. After ORIF, 5–8 weeks is usually all that is required for resumption of sport.

## 2.4 Hook of the Hamate Fracture

### 2.4.1 Clinical Presentation

Fracture of the hamate can occur while swinging a golf club, tennis racquet, or baseball bat. The fracture is especially likely to happen when the golf club strikes the ground instead of the ball, forcing the top of the handle of the club against the hook of the hamate. This mechanism may also compress the terminal branches of the ulnar nerve, producing sensory and motor changes. As a result, patient symptoms include reduced grip strength, numbness and tingling in the distribution of the ulnar nerve, as well as ulnar sided wrist pain.

### 2.4.2 Diagnosis

Hamate fractures may go undiagnosed until there is rupture of the long flexor tendon of the small finger. Early examination reveals tenderness over the hook of the hamate. Swelling may or may not be prominent. Plain x-rays of the wrist do not image the fracture. Instead, carpal tunnel views with the wrist in dorsiflexion or an ulnar oblique view must be ordered.

### 2.4.3 Treatment

The hook of the hamate is the point of attachment for hypothenar muscles, and when fractured through the base, these muscles alternately stress the fracture in different directions, predisposing to nonunion. As a result, this fracture rarely heals with immobilization. Surgical removal of the fractured hook followed by 3 weeks of wrist immobilization is usually required. After this, a comprehensive rehabilitation program is undergone to restore full mobility and function.

### 2.4.4 Return to Play

Assuming no complications and proper healing, sport can resume 6 weeks after surgery.

## 2.5 Distal Radius Fracture

Distal radius fractures are the most common forearm fracture. Etiology usually involves a fall on an outstretched hand, although different subsets of this fracture group may have slightly different etiologies. Classification of distal radius fractures is based on angulation, displacement, intra- or extra-articular injury, and ulnar or carpal bone involvement. Terms included within the term of distal radius fracture include Colles' fracture, Smith's fracture, Barton's fracture, and Chaffeur's fracture. These names are applied to specific patterns of fracture. The Colles' fracture is reported to be the most common distal radial fracture. Specifically it refers to radial fracture in the distal 2 cm of the bone with dorsal displacement. An ulnar styloid fracture may or may not be present.

### 2.5.1  Universal Classification of Distal Radius Fracture

1. Nonarticular, nondisplaced
2. Nonarticular displaced

   a. Reducible, stable
   b. Reducible, unstable
   c. Irreducible

3. Articular, nondisplaced
4. Articular, displaced

   a. Reducible, stable
   b. Reducible, unstable
   c. Irreducible
   d. Complex

### 2.5.2  Clinical Presentation

The most common history provided with regard to this injury is a fall on an out-stretched hand with considerable force. The patient usually notes tenderness and swelling at the wrist.

### 2.5.3  Diagnosis

Deformity, swelling, tenderness, and loss of wrist range of motion are features of an exam when a distal radius fracture is present. Posteroanterior (PA), lateral, and oblique radiographs of the injured forearm should be obtained. Oblique views reveal intra-articular involvement not apparent on the other views. The examiner should note the direction of displacement, angulation, degree of comminution, presence of intra-articular involvement, and radial length or variance as compared with the unaffected side.

### 2.5.4  Treatment

Management of a distal radius fracture involves anesthetizing the affected area and placing the arm in traction to unlock any fragments. The deformity is then reduced with a closed reduction and casted. X-ray is used to ensure that the reduction was successful. It should be noted that maintaining good position in adults is particularly difficult and serial imaging is required. If callus is seen on x-ray at 3 weeks, the cast can be replaced with a removable splint. Many orthopedic surgeons favor a more extended period of 6 weeks in a cast even in the presence of callus formation. After cast removal a period of rehabilitation is required to allow for recovery of strength and ROM. Failure of casting is common and has a large risk of an adverse outcome. Studies have shown that the fracture often re-displaces to its original position in a cast. Long term this increases the risk of stiffness and osteoarthritis, leading to long-term wrist pain and loss of function. Given these findings, surgical interventions such as open reduction internal fixation (ORIF), external fixation, or percutaneous pinning are indicated at times.

### 2.5.5 Return to Play

Prognosis and return to play correlate with severity of injury, with a nondisplaced extra-articular fracture having a better prognosis than an unstable, displaced intra-articular fracture. If managed with a cast, time course to return of play is largely dependent on healing. Those with nondisplaced fractures may be able to return to play not long after injury with a protective splint. In order to be a candidate for return, the patient should exhibit early signs of healing on imaging and no pain. Obviously, additional precautions must be taken for those participating in contact sports and deferment of play for at least a few weeks is advisable. After ORIF, athletes may return to play with protection at as little as 3 weeks. This time is increased to 6 weeks if the fracture was displaced. A patient should never return to play if strength and function are not adequate to prevent reinjury.

## 2.6   Carpal Tunnel Syndrome

Carpal tunnel syndrome (CTS) is a compression neuropathy of the median nerve. Although compression of the median nerve can occur at multiple levels, CTS refers to compression at the wrist by the transverse carpal ligament.

### 2.6.1   Clinical Presentation

The degree of symptoms depends on the chronicity and degree of compression. Symptoms can progress from purely sensory to include motor loss with associated atrophy. Sensation loss occurs at the tips of the first three fingers and may travel to the forearm and wrist. Weakness of grip may occur in more advanced cases. Patients typically state that symptoms are worst at night or after participating in a repetitive activity.

### 2.6.2   Diagnosis

History and physical exam are highly suggestive of the diagnosis of CTS. Sensation should be tested in the median nerve distribution, as should the strength of thumb opposition. Provocative tests include Tinel's sign and Phalen's sign (Fig. 7.2). Tinel's sign involves tapping over the transverse carpal ligament with the wrist held

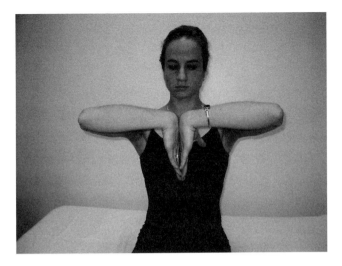

**Fig. 7.2** Phalen's sign

in extension. Phalen's sign involves holding both wrists in extreme volar flexion for 30–60 seconds. Electromyography (EMG) and nerve conduction velocity (NCV) studies can be performed to confirm clinical suspicion. NCV testing is positive in approximately 70% of cases. It should be noted that a negative NCV does not exclude the possibility of median nerve compression. If symptoms are intermittent and mild, NCV/EMG may be normal. In these cases, a median nerve block can be used to confirm the diagnosis.

### 2.6.3 Treatment

Mild to moderate CTS can be managed medically, whereas advanced CTS requires surgical release. Medical management includes minimizing provocative factors. This might require reducing gripping, grasping, or repetitive wrist motion. A Velcro wrist splint with a metal stay to reduce symptoms is also recommended. At the least, the splint should be used at night. When indicated, a steroid injection can be highly useful. Corticosteroid injection is advanced just through the transverse carpal tunnel ligament to bathe the nerve and relieve inflammation. Many patients have good relief after one injection.

### 2.6.4 Return to Play

Those suffering from CTS can participate in sport as tolerated. Splints as described in the treatment section may assist avoiding aggravating factors.

## 2.7 Ulnar Nerve Palsy (Handlebar Palsy)

Handlebar palsy is a common problem for competitive and recreational cyclists. Compression is the result of direct pressure on the ulnar nerve from grip on the handlebars. Often, the nerve may be stretched or hyperextended when a drop-down handlebar is held in the lower position. Due to the change of riding position and shape of handlebars (horn handle) in recent years, a single bicycle ride may be sufficient to cause disruption of the ulnar branch. This is especially relevant in downhill riding when a large part of the body weight is supported by the hand on the corner of the handlebar leading to a high load at Guyon's canal.

### 2.7.1   Clinical Presentation

The ulnar nerve controls sensation in the ring and little finger and controls most of the muscular function of the hand. The pressure placed on the ulnar nerve results in numbness and tingling in the ring and little finger or hand weakness, or a combination of both.

### 2.7.2   Diagnosis

Diagnosis is made largely on the basis of the history and physical exam. Suspicion can be confirmed by performing EMG/NCV studies.

### 2.7.3   Treatment

Symptoms can take from several days to months to resolve, but surgical treatment is rarely necessary. Rest, stretching exercises, and anti-inflammatory medications usually help relieve the symptoms. Applying less pressure or weight to the handlebars and avoiding hyperextension can help to prevent a recurrence. Other advisable changes include padded gloves, wrist splints, and adjusting the position of the hands on the handlebar.

### 2.7.4   Return to Play

Those suffering from ulnar neuropathy can participate in sport as tolerated. However, adjustments should be made to reduce the risk of reinjury.

## 2.8 Metacarpophalangeal Instability (Gamekeeper's Thumb, Skier's Thumb)

Injury to the thumb ligament is one of the most common skiing injuries. It ranks second only to knee sprains. Skier's thumb is a strain or tear to the thumb's major stabilizing ligament—the ulnar collateral ligament of the MCP joint of the thumb. The ulnar collateral ligament assists in grasping, pinching, and stabilizing items in the hand.

### 2.8.1 Clinical Presentation

Injury to the thumb while skiing usually results from a fall on an outstretched hand that continues to hold the ski pole. At impact, the thumb is driven directly into the snow and is bent back or to the side, away from the palm and index finger, straining or tearing the ligament. When injured, the ulnar collateral ligament cannot support the thumb, making grasping or pinching with the thumb difficult. Patients complain of pain and swelling along the ulnar aspect of the MP joint. This initial complaint of pain may progress to weakness or instability.

### 2.8.2 Diagnosis

Valgus stress determines the laxity of the ulnar collateral ligament. An incomplete rupture is characterized by <30 degrees of laxity or <15 degrees more laxity than in the uninjured thumb. A complete rupture is characterized by >30 degrees of laxity or >5 degrees than the uninjured thumb. X-rays should be performed to rule out avulsion. In the absence of avulsion, x-rays are negative. MRI can be performed to determine the relationship of the torn ligament in relation to its surrounding muscles. This may be useful if surgery is required.

### 2.8.3 Treatment

Referral to an orthopedist or hand surgeon is indicated when x-ray shows an avulsed fragment >11 mm displaced from its origin. Referral is also appropriate for those with complete ligament tears determined by physical exam. For nonsurgical candidates, ice should be immediately applied to the effected area. A dorsal hood or thumb spica splint is used to immobilize the joint for at least 3 to 5 weeks. To avoid injury, skiers can use strapless poles. A better protective measure is to advise skiers to discard poles when they fall. This will prevent radial deviation of the thumb upon impact. For an already injured thumb, gloves that have built-in splints can be used.

### 2.8.4 Return to Play

After an incomplete injury, the thumb must remain completely protected for 3 weeks, after which gentle ROM exercises can begin. If surgical repair is necessary, a minimum of 2 weeks of rest should be recommended.

Heavy lifting or gripping should be avoided until grip strength has returned to normal.

## 2.9 Metacarpal Shaft/Neck Fracture

Injury to the metacarpals is varied in etiology. Usually the fractures are classified according to pathology (transverse, oblique, or spiral). The fracture pattern tends to correlate with injury mechanism. Direct or axial injury results in a transverse or oblique fracture, whereas torsional force tends to cause spiral fractures. Fractures of the fifth metacarpal neck are among the most common hand fractures and are most often associated with striking a solid object with a closed fist. Although these fractures have been nicknamed "boxer's fractures" they rarely occur during boxing. A skilled fighter is more likely to fracture the index metacarpal given that this is along the greatest line of force when throwing a punch with correct form.

### 2.9.1  Clinical Presentation

Fracture of the metacarpal is usually a result of force applied to a clenched fist or a direct blow to the hand. A patient will usually give a history consistent with such an injury. Pain and swelling are typical complaints. The patient may also note asymmetry of the knuckles.

### 2.9.2  Diagnosis

Metacarpal fractures are easily diagnosed by localized tenderness and swelling on physical exam. In addition, there is loss of the normal contour of the dorsum of the finger. Ecchymosis on the palmar surface is highly suggestive of fracture. X-ray confirms what is clinically suspected.

### 2.9.3  Treatment

Treatment of metacarpal fractures focuses on reduction when necessary and splinting. Splints should be forearm based and allow motion of the IP joint. They should extend over the dorsal and palmar aspect of the entire effected metacarpal. Generally, the wrist should be placed in 20–30 degrees of extension and the MCP joint immobilized in 70–90 degrees of flexion. Buddy taping the fingers can aid in maintaining some degree of rotational control. After a short period of immobilization, patients should be encouraged to use the affected finger. With regard to metacarpal shaft fractures, only small amounts of angulation are acceptable. The exact degree is dependent on the digit involved. The more proximal the fracture the more pronounced the deformity and the less angulation that can be accepted. All malrotation must be addressed surgically. Metacarpal neck fractures can tolerate a larger degree of angulation (50–60 degrees). Rarely does a neck fracture require surgery. Open fractures always require operative débridement and irrigation followed by stable internal or external fixation. The patient should be monitored throughout the healing process with serial imaging to assure proper positioning.

### 2.9.4  Return to Play

Immobilization does not usually extend beyond 4 weeks. At this time, there is usually evidence of healing on imaging. After this period of initial immobilization, an orthotic should be used for an additional 4–6 weeks when participating in sports.

## 2.10  Baseball Finger (Mallet Finger)

Baseball finger is caused by sudden passive flexion of the extended DIP joint causing rupture of the extensor tendon. It is also known as baseball finger because it can occur when a finger is jammed while catching a ball.

### 2.10.1  Clinical Presentation

Clinically, the DIP joint is flexed and cannot be actively extended. The patient may give a history of a ball "jamming" the finger.

### 2.10.2  Diagnosis

Mallet finger is diagnosed by physical examination. On exam, the patient is asked to actively extend the finger tip. If the last joint cannot be straightened actively, then a mallet finger diagnosis is appropriate. Other signs of mallet finger on exam include swelling and tenderness around the fingertip. An x-ray may be indicated to rule out avulsion if clinically suspected.

### 2.10.3  Treatment

Conservative treatment involves splinting of the DIP in extension for 6–8 weeks with a Stack splint. Position should be checked weekly to prevent contracture formation. For the 2 weeks following initial splinting, gentle active flexion and nightly splinting should be performed. If healing is poor or there is an avulsed fragment, then surgical treatment may be indicated.

### 2.10.4  Return to Play

If the splint is worn as indicated, activity can be resumed immediately. Obviously, certain sports are more risky than others with regard to re-injury and a decision to return to play must be made on a case-by-case basis. Not seeking medical attention immediately after injury and failing to allow complete healing can lead to permanent injury or deformity of the hand.

## 2.11 Trigger Finger (Flexor Tenosynovitis)

Trigger finger is an inflammation of the flexor tendon sheath of the finger. The flexor tendons for each digit course through a sheath located between the metacarpal and distal interphalangeal joint. Specifically, the flexor digitorum superficialis attaches to the middle phalanges and the flexor digitorum profundus attaches to the distal phalanges. Repetitive trauma can cause inflammation of the flexor tendon and sheaths at the metacarpophalangeal joint. The resultant abnormal gliding impairs the flexion pulley system and ultimately forms a nodule in the tendon. As the digit flexes, the nodule passes under the pulley system and gets caught on the annular sheath, locking the finger in a flexed position.

### 2.11.1 Clinical Presentation

Patients often complain of pain and snapping when they move the affected digit. They may complain of a locking of the finger in the flexed position.

### 2.11.2 Diagnosis

Diagnosis is based on history and physical exam. On exam, there is tenderness at the base of the finger. Clicking or locking with flexion may be noted. In addition, a nodule may be felt at the base of the finger. A local anesthetic block can be used to confirm diagnosis but is rarely necessary.

### 2.11.3 Treatment

Conservative treatment involves NSAIDs and steroid injection as well as physical therapy. All of these interventions reduce swelling of the tendon, allowing it to glide freely in and out of the sheath. A single injection is all that is needed in 50% of cases. A further 25% will respond to a second injection (i.e., three fourths of patients can be successfully treated in this way). Injection causes no general side effects but occasionally the skin around the injection site can be thinned by the steroid; therefore, two injections are the maximum. Surgery may be indicated if steroid injections do not work. It involves a small procedure under local anesthetic during which a slit is made in the mouth of the sheath to prevent the tendon catching at this point.

### 2.11.4 Return to Play

After injection, the finger should be rested for three days. Following this initial period of rest, the fingers can be used but in a protected manger (buddy tape) for the next 3–4 weeks. Repetitive grasping, gripping and vibration should be avoided.

## 2.12 Jersey Finger

Jersey finger is an injury to the flexor digitorum profundus or superficialis tendon resulting in an inability to bend a fingertip. The common action in all injuries is extension of the finger against resistance. This is most often noted in athletes who grab one another's jerseys. Strain, rupture, or avulsion occurs when the jersey is pulled from the athlete's finger. The ring finger is the most commonly involved digit because of its limited independent extensibility.

### 2.12.1 Clinical Presentation

Patients usually complain of pain when moving the injured finger and an inability to bend the last joint. A pop or rip may have been felt in the finger at the time of injury.

### 2.12.2 Diagnosis

Diagnosis is based largely on history and physical exam. The finger can be bent forward passively but not actively and a lump may be felt in the palm or finger. After 48 hours, there is usually some bruising. X-rays will rule out an associated fracture.

### 2.12.3 Treatment

The initial phase of rest, ice, and elevation is usually followed by surgery, and then a graduated program of stretching and strengthening. In the months following surgery it is especially important to concentrate on increasing the endurance of the injured area's muscles to help prevent re-injury. One often neglected part of rehabilitation involves re-training proprioception in the injured area. This has been shown to help reduce the incidence of re-injury.

### 2.12.4 Return to Play

Return to sports is usually not recommended for at least 3 months after surgery.

# Reference

1. Slaby FJ, McCune SK, Summers RW (1994) Gross anatomy in the practice of medicine, 1st edn. Lippincott Williams & Wilkins, Baltimore

# Chapter 8
# Lower Back Injuries

Grant Cooper, Joseph E. Herrera, and Michael Dambeck

## 1 Introduction

Low back pain is a common, debilitating problem for athletes as well as the general population. It is the number one cause for athletes to miss a professional sporting event. Most cases of lower back pain are self-limiting, lasting no more than a few weeks. Occasionally, however, back pain lasts longer than 3 months, at which point it is termed chronic back pain.

There are many potential pain generators in the lower back. The discs, facet joints, sacroiliac joint, bones, ligaments, muscles, tendons, and soft tissues can all cause pain. In younger athletes who have axial back pain with trunk flexion, the disc is often suspected as the potential underlying cause. Younger athletes with pain on extension may be suspected of having a pars interarticularis fracture. Older patients may be more likely to have facet joint disease as an underlying cause, particularly if their pain is more extension based. Of course, these are very broad brush strokes and are just meant to keep in the back of your mind to give you a framework within which to work. Each athlete must naturally be treated as an individual and interrogated appropriately. This chapter is aimed to help guide you along that path.

## 2 Anatomy

The vertebrae increase in size distally, with the lumbar vertebrae being the largest. Each lumbar vertebra consists of a body, spinous process, two transverse processes, pedicles, laminae, and the superior and inferior articular processes. In between each vertebra is an intervertebral disc that acts as a shock absorber. The lumbar functional unit is composed of two vertebral bodies, the intervertebral disc, and the associated posterior elements. Several intraspinal ligaments surround the spinal unit to assist in stabilization. Together, this unit transmits loads from one vertebra to the next and allows flexion-extension movements to take place, provide stability, and prevent translatory and torsional shear. Seventy-five percent of lumbar flexion and extension occurs at the lumbosacral spine, 20% at L4-L5, and 5% at the other levels.

J.E. Herrera and G. Cooper (eds.), *Essential Sports Medicine*,
doi: 10.1007/978-1-59745-414-8, © Humana Press 2008

The anterior longitudinal ligament extends along the anterior aspects of the vertebrae, whereas the posterior longitudinal ligament extends along the posterior aspects. The two help maintain the axial stability of the spinal column. The anterior segment of the spine has a weight-bearing and shock-absorbing component, whereas the posterior segment helps protect the neural structures.

The intervertebral disc may be thought of as similar to a jelly donut that also functions as a shock absorber. It is made up of the nucleus pulposus and annulus fibrosus. The nucleus pulposus is the gelatinous center of the disc that can be thought of as the jelly portion of the donut. The annulus fibrosus is the tough collagenous ring that surrounds the nucleus. Within the outer third of the annulus fibrosus, there are nerve fibers capable of transmitting pain signals to the brain. When the disc is the source of pain, it is because a tear has occurred in the annulus and these nerve fibers have become irritated. A tear in the annulus, as will be discussed later in the chapter, does not necessarily have to coincide with a bulging disc.

# 3  Lower Back Injuries

## 3.1  Lumbar Sprain and Strain

A strain is a muscular injury in which muscle fibers have been torn. This is typically a result of overstretching. A sprain is an injury to the ligament in which the ligament is overstretched and fibers are torn. Minor tearing of a ligament is considered a first degree sprain. A complete tear of a ligament is a third degree sprain. Any muscle or ligament in the body can undergo a sprain/strain, respectively. The back is replete with muscles and ligaments and because of the torques and compressive forces that the back undergoes, sprains and strains are common in athletes.

### 3.1.1  Clinical Presentation

Patients typically present with a history of a minor pain while participating in an activity. For example, a softball player may report feeling a "twinge" in his back while throwing a ball. Then, later that night the discomfort may increase. When the patient wakes up the next day, the pain may have worsened. He may feel a spasm in his back. The pain may radiate into the buttock but rarely will radiate beneath the knee. The pain will be aggravated by movement and made better by rest. After 24–48 hours, the pain generally starts getting better, although it may not completely heal for 1–3 weeks.

### 3.1.2  Diagnosis

On physical examination, the patient will have tenderness over the affected area. The neurological examination should be normal. Imaging studies are not necessary unless being obtained to rule out another pathology.

### 3.1.3 Treatment

PRICE (protection, rest, ice, compression, elevation) is the treatment. The patient should have relative rest. This means he or she should "take it easy" and not over-exert, but also not stay in bed 24 hours a day. Movement helps keep the back limber and the blood flowing. Ice is an excellent anti-inflammatory agent. A bag of peas is a good ice substitute. Ice should be applied for 20 minutes four times per day. Over-the-counter anti-inflammatory medication can also be used.

Physical therapy is also a good adjunctive treatment. Although not necessary to get over the acute injury, once a person has suffered one back sprain or strain, he or she is more likely to suffer another one. A good physical therapy program that teaches the patient a home exercise program to achieve lumbar stabilization and limb flexibility will help the patient avoid future injury.

### 3.1.4 Return to Sport

Once the patient is pain free with full range of motion, he or she may return to sport. It is a good idea for the patient to have gone to a physical therapist prior to return to sport and have begun an exercise program to strengthen the core and improve body biomechanics to help avoid future injury.

## 3.2 Spondylolysis and Spondylolisthesis

One of the most common causes of lower back pain in the young athlete involves a stress fracture of the pars interarticularis. The pars interarticularis is stressed with lumbar extension. Athletes who participate in activities involving repetitive extension (e.g., gymnasts, ballet dancers, divers, baseball pitchers) are at increased risk to suffer a pars stress fracture. Once a pars fracture has occurred, particularly if it occurs bilaterally, the athlete may go on to develop a spondylolisthesis. This is when one vertebral body moves in relation to the adjacent one. The degree of spondylolisthesis can be graded (Table 8.1).

More than 80% of cases of spondylolisthesis are caused by a pars fracture (isthmic spondylolisthesis) and occur at the L5-S1 level. About 10% of the remaining cases occur at the L4-L5 level.

An important note is that many young athletes may have *asymptomatic* pars stress fractures. About 7% of asymptomatic 18-year-old people have radiographic evidence of pars stress fractures.

**Table 8.1** Spondylolisthesis grading

| |
|---|
| Grade 1: 0–24% slippage |
| Grade 2: 25–50% slippage |
| Grade 3: 51–75% slippage |
| Grade 4: >75% slippage |

### 3.2.1   Clinical Presentation

Patients may complain of a history of mild lower back pain that has become worse and progressive to the point that participating in activities that require lumbar extension is not tolerated. Often, the patient may report participation in gymnastics, swimming, football, or soccer. The pain may refer to the buttocks and posterior thighs.

Rarely, if the patient has a spondylolisthesis that is compressing a nerve root or creating central canal stenosis, symptoms of shooting pain, numbness, and/or burning may be present in the lower extremities.

### 3.2.2   Diagnosis

Physical examination may not reveal any bony tenderness. Muscle spasms may overlie the affected bony structures. Pain is typically worsened with trunk extension and oblique extension. The single leg hyperextension test (Stork test) is often useful (Fig. 8.1). In this test, if the patient has right sided back pain, he or she stands on the right leg and leans in lumbar oblique extension over the right leg. This is

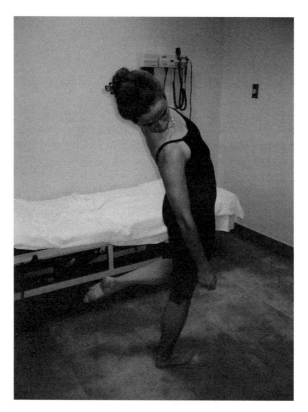

**Fig. 8.1** Stork test

considered the most sensitive physical exam maneuver to detect a pars interarticularis stress fracture.

In patients with a spondylolisthesis of grade II or higher, a step-off may be present on palpation between vertebrae. If the spondylolisthesis is creating nerve root involvement, weakness, numbness, and reflex involvement may be found in the distribution of the involved nerves.

X-rays often reveal the presence of a pars fracture. Lumbar AP and lateral x-rays will show the presence of a spondylolisthesis and may indicate the presence of a fracture, but oblique films are needed to adequately visualize the pars. Oblique films should be gotten with caution, however, because they require considerably more radiation than AP and lateral films. Even with oblique films, plain films may not reveal the presence of a fracture. If clinical suspicion is high, a bone scan with SPECT may be helpful. This will only light up over the pars if the fracture is present and active.

If a radiculopathy is suspected, an MRI is useful to obtain to evaluate the site and degree of nerve root compression.

### 3.2.3  Treatment

In patients with acute spondylolysis, bracing and rest are appropriate first line treatments. In these patients, a bone scan should confirm the presence of an active acute lesion. A Boston overlapping brace, lumbar corset, or warm-n-form orthosis, is used to prevent hyperextension. The brace is typically worn for 23 hours per day until the patient is asymptomatic for 3 months. At that time, a repeat bone scan with SPECT should be obtained. Physical therapy regimens should emphasize hamstring stretching and lumbar flexibility while using the brace. In patients with persistent pain despite aggressive conservative care, medial branch blocks may be performed under fluoroscopic guidance to confirm the diagnosis. If the diagnosis is confirmed, rhizotomy of the medial branches supplying the involved facet joint may relieve the symptoms.

Patients with spondylolisthesis and nerve root impingement may be candidates for epidural steroid injections. Flexion and extension radiographs of the spine may be necessary to check for any potential instability. Progressive neurological symptoms and/or change in bowel or bladder function require urgent surgical evaluation.

### 3.2.4  Return to Play

In general, athletes are able to return to play when they are pain free throughout the entire ROM regardless of whether or not there is radiographic healing.

## 3.3  Radiculopathy and "Disc Herniation"

The intervertebral disc sits between the vertebral bodies and serves as a shock absorber between the bones. For a disc to cause pain, it does *not* have to bulge or herniate. It just has to have a tear in the annulus fibrosus. In fact, a painful disc may look perfectly normal on MRI. A disc herniation, then, is not synonymous or even necessarily related to discogenic back pain. (Of course, the two may and often do coexist.) A disc bulge or herniation refers to when the disc moves out from its physiological place in the spine. When this happens, it may compress a nerve root and cause pain, numbness, and/or tingling radiating down the lower extremity, as well as potentially weakness. Macnab classified the degree of disc herniation (Table 8.2).

### 3.3.1  Clinical Presentation

A typical patient will complain of pain radiating down the buttock into the lower extremity. For example, a 26-year-old football player felt a sudden dull pain in his left buttock that radiated down the outside of his leg following a tackle. The pain subsided but after the game he noticed it returned. Over the last 8 days, he says the pain has gotten much worse. He says the pain has become a sharp pain in his lower back that radiates into his buttock and down the lateral thigh into the lateral calf, foot, and big toe. He complains of mild numbness in his lateral calf but says the rest of the pain feels more "electric" and "shooting" in nature. Leaning forward and sitting for a prolonged period of time makes the symptoms worse.

If the symptoms are severe or prolonged, a patient may also complain of weakness. Depending on the level of nerve being impinged by the disc, the distribution of symptoms will be different (Table 8.3).

### 3.3.2  Diagnosis

On physical examination, numbness, weakness, and diminished reflexes may be found in the distribution of the affected nerve root. A positive slump test (Fig. 8.2) and straight leg raise may also be positive. If the L2 or L3 nerve root are involved, a reverse straight leg raise may be positive.

If a Babinski sign is found or reflexes are hyperactive and asymmetrical, suspicion for cord impingement should be raised and addressed urgently.

AP and lateral x-rays may be obtained to evaluate the bony structures. However, some physicians choose to just get an MRI without the x-rays, which is the best test

---

**Table 8.2**  Macnab's classification

*Bulging Disc*: A bulge and convexity of the disc, but with an intact annulus fibrosus
*Prolapsed Disc*: Disc herniates posteriorly through an incomplete defect in the annulus fibrosus
*Extruded Disc*: Disc herniates posteriorly through a complete defect in the annulus fibrosus
*Sequestered Disc*: A portion of the nucleus pulposus extrudes through a complete defect in the annulus fibrosus and has lost continuity with the nucleus pulposus.

Depalma M (2006) Nonspondylolytic etiologies of lumbar pain in the young athlete. Curr Sports Med Repts 5:44–49

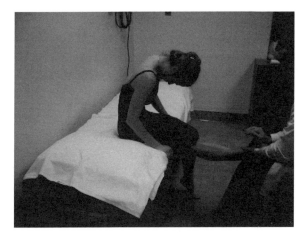

**Fig. 8.2** Slump test

in this situation to evaluate the degree and level of impingement. If an MRI is contraindicated, CT is another option.

### 3.3.3 Treatment

Conservative care includes RICE (as outlined under the Sprain and Strain section). Physical therapy to focus on core stabilization should also be started. Exercises should be extension based to reduce the pressure on the disc. Anti-inflammatory medication may be helpful also.

If symptoms persist, or if symptoms are particularly severe, an epidural steroid injection under fluoroscopic guidance should be considered. An oral steroid taper can also be considered, although there are more systemic side effects with this approach and the medication does not get as close to the actual source of inflammation when compared with an epidural injection.

If the patient presents with progressive neurological deficits, or the patient has bladder incontinence or saddle anesthesia, emergent MRI and surgical evaluation is needed.

### 3.3.4 Return to Sport

Once the patient is pain free with full ROM, he or she may return to sport. However, as with other conditions, it is advisable that the patient learn improved postural biomechanics and implement a home exercise program of core stabilization and stretching to help prevent future injury prior to return to sport.

## 3.4   Internal Disc Disruption

As has been discussed, the nerve fibers in the disc are present in the outer third of the annulus. There have been limited reports of these fibers extending into the middle third of the annulus. For a disc to cause pain there must be irritation of these fibers by a tear in the annulus. Once there is an annular tear, mechanical pressures as well as chemical irritation from inflammatory substances within the nucleus pulposus leads to back pain. X-rays may reveal decreased disc space, but they may be normal. An MRI may reveal a high intensity zone (HIZ) in the posterior disc, but the MRI may also be normal. There is currently no imaging study that can reliably diagnose discogenic back pain.

### 3.4.1   Clinical Presentation

Patients typically complain of dull, achy back pain. The pain may have started during a flexion exercise. For example, a rugby player experienced a sudden pain in his lower back while performing a squat in the gym. He says the pain is worse with flexion and sitting. The pain is worse in the morning and better with walking. Disc pain is typically worse in the morning because pressure in the disc rises over night secondary to gravity as well as hormonal factors.

The pain may refer into the buttock but rarely extends into the lower extremities beyond the knees.

### 3.4.2   Diagnosis

Acute disc pain may present similarly to a lower back strain or sprain. Indeed, if the pain improves after a week or two, it is unlikely that the physician or patient will know if the cause was a strain or sprain or an annular tear. However, if the pain persists beyond 1 month, it is unlikely that the cause is a simple sprain/strain without an underlying cause. In this instance, or if the pain is particularly severe, more aggressive diagnosis is needed. X-rays and MRI may be suggestive of discogenic pain. However, the gold standard for diagnosis remains a provocative lumbar discography. In this procedure, a needle is inserted under fluoroscopic guidance into the disc and dye is injected. If the patient's pain is reproduced at one level under low pressure injection and not at other disc levels, the painful disc is the cause of pain.

### 3.4.3   Treatment

Initial treatment consists of RICE and physical therapy, focusing on lumbar stabilization and stretching. If pain persists, intradiscal electrothermal annuloplasty (IDET) is another treatment option in younger patients with well preserved disc spaces. This is a percutaneous procedure in which a catheter is introduced into the annulus of the disc and the annulus is heated up, denaturing the collagen as well as the nerve fibers. In this patient population, with confirmed disc pain, IDET has about a 75 % success rate according to some studies. If pain is persistent and disabling, disc replacement or fusion surgery should be considered as a last resort.

### 3.4.4   Return to Sport

Pain free range of motion is required. A home exercise program for lumbar stabilization and stretching should be instituted to reduce the risk of future injury.

## 3.5   Sacroiliac Joint Pain

The sacroiliac joint is believed to be the source of up to 10% of chronic lower back pain. In sports, with the repetitive movement and torsional forces placed on the spine, the sacroiliac joint suffers repetitive stress and this may predispose to injury. It is thought that in addition to repetitive stress, sacroiliac joint pain may be due to muscle imbalances.

### 3.5.1   Clinical Presentation

The typical patient is a young athlete who presents with a dull, achy pain over the sacrum. The patient may be a young woman who was participating in dance class. Following class, she noted soreness in her lower back that did not go away. After a week of persistent soreness, she presented to the doctor. Typically, patients do not have radiating pain into the lower extremities. However, dull, achy referral pain patterns may extend into the buttocks. Pain is worse with activity and better with rest.

### 3.5.2   Diagnosis

On physical examination, the FABERE test may be positive (Fig. 8.3). In this test, the patient's ankle is placed onto the contralateral knee. The examiner then places a compressive force onto the flexed knee as well as the contralateral anterior sacroiliac spine (ASIS).

X-rays and MRI may be obtained but are not generally helpful in diagnosing this condition, but they may exclude other conditions. The gold standard for diagnosing sacroiliac joint pain is to inject anesthetic and cortisone into the joint under fluoroscopic guidance. When this relieves the patient's pain, the sacroiliac joint is believed to be the underlying cause.

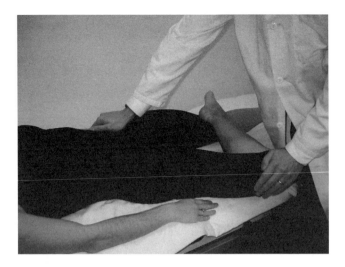

**Fig. 8.3** FABERE test

### 3.5.3   Treatment

PRICE and physical therapy are first-line treatments. Physical therapy focuses on stretching and strengthening exercises, core stabilization, and correcting any potential muscle imbalances. Sacroiliac joint steroid injections performed under fluoroscopic guidance may also be helpful. Sacroiliac joint belts also may provide symptom relief.

### 3.5.4   Return to Sport

The patient may return to sport once he or she has full, pain free ROM.

## 3.6   Facet Joint Syndrome

The facet joints in the back are paired synovial joints. They allow the spine to flex and extend and help prevent anterior and posterior displacement. Trunk extension and oblique extension in particular loads the facet joints. Just like any other synovial joint (e.g., knee), the facet joints can become arthritic and painful. In fact, as much as 40% of chronic lower back pain in older individuals, and 20% of younger individuals is thought to be due to facet joint disease. Sports that involved repetitive trunk extension (e.g., tennis, throwing sports, swimming, gymnastics) may predispose to facet joint disease.

### 3.6.1 Clinical Presentation

Typically, patients present with complaints of gradually progressive lower back pain that is worse with extension and made better with sitting. The pain may refer into the lower extremities but rarely extends beneath the knees. If the facet joints have hypertrophied and are impinging a nerve root, the patient may complain of radicular symptoms.

### 3.6.2 Diagnosis

On physical examination, the patient will often have pain that is worse with trunk extension and oblique extension (Fig. 8.4). The Stork test may be positive. If a nerve root is impinged, findings of radiculopathy may be present. Otherwise, the neurological examination should be normal.

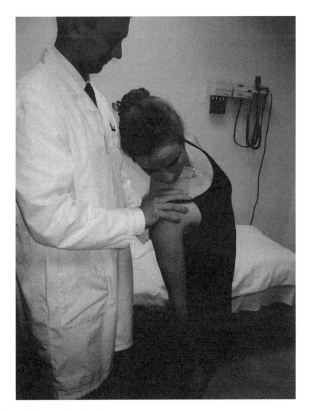

**Fig. 8.4** Lumbar oblique extension

X-rays may reveal facet arthropathy. MRI may also reveal arthritic changes in the joint. However, neither x-ray nor MRI can reliably diagnose facet joint pain. Recently, bone scan with SPECT has been used with some success to make the diagnosis. However, as with many other spinal conditions, the gold standard diagnosis remains diagnostic blocks of the facet joints. The facet joint can be blocked with medial branch blocks in which a small amount of anesthetic medication is placed onto the medial branch nerve that supplies the facet. Alternatively, an intra-articular facet joint injection can be performed. These injections are performed under fluoroscopic guidance. The advantage of the intra-articular injection is that it has the potential to be therapeutic as well as diagnostic. Ideally, because facet joint blocks have about a 25% false-positive rate, double blind blocks should be performed.

### 3.6.3   Treatment

RICE and physical therapy that focuses on flexion-based lumbar stabilization exercises can be very effective. Oral anti-inflammatory medication can also be helpful. When these interventions are not effective, intra-articular injections of the involved facet joints can be helpful. Unfortunately, physical examination is unreliable for predicting *which* facet joints are likely involved and so multiple levels may need to be injected. If intra-articular injections provide only short-term relief, percutaneous rhizotomy of the medial branches with radiofrequency is very effective in providing pain relief for patients with facet joint pain. This procedure essentially burns the medial branches, cutting the communicating signal of pain from the facet joint to the brain. The nerves regenerate over time, however, and the pain may return. The procedure may need to be repeated every 6 months to 2 years.

### 3.6.4   Return to Sport

The patient should exhibit full and pain-free range of motion. The patient should be involved in a structured home exercise program to focus on core stabilization with flexion bias and stretching.

## 3.7   Transverse Process Fracture

Fractures in the lumbar spine are rare in sports medicine. The spine can be conveniently divided into three sections based on Denis classification. For a fracture to create instability, it must involve two columns. A transverse process fracture takes place in the posterior column and is thus stable. This type of fracture typically results from lateral bending and/or rotation.

### 3.7.1   Clinical Presentation

The typical patient will relate a history of trauma. For example, the patient may be a young skateboarder who fell from a height while twisting in the air and suffered immediate back pain. Or, the patient may be a football player who got tackled by a helmet in the back (spearing, which is a penalty). Although a transverse process fracture is not considered to be serious in long-term considerations, they are exquisitely painful in the short term (similar to a broken rib).

### 3.7.2   Diagnosis

The diagnosis of this type of fracture is based on plain films. If the fracture is not clear on plain films, the diagnosis can be confirmed with a bone scan.

### 3.7.3   Treatment

Rest and pain control is the first step of treatment. The patient should be advised to modify activity until pain is controlled. Bracing is rarely used.

### 3.7.4   Return to Sport

The patient may return to full participation when strength and pain free range of motion are restored.

## 3.8   *Compression Fracture*

Traumatic compression fractures occur when there is significant axial or essentially vertical load injury with anterior or lateral flexion causing failure of the anterior column. The middle column remains intact and may act as a hinge. These fractures are usually stable. It is rare for these fractures to involve neurological compromise.

### 3.8.1   Clinical Presentation

The patient will usually recall the traumatic event that involved significant axial loading on the spine. Typically this occurs during landing following a high jump in gymnastics, or a head on tackle in football. The patient will complain of stiffness of the trunk and localized pain.

### 3.8.2   Diagnosis

The patient will present with pain and stiffness on trunk movement with decreased ROM and localized pain on palpation. The fracture can be identified on AP and lateral x-rays. Flexion and extension views, as well as CT scan can be used to determine the stability of the fracture.

### 3.8.3   Treatment

Treatment is usually conservative, with rest and pain control being the initial goals. Patients may need to wear a brace to help alleviate pain. When the patient is pain free, physical therapy with focus on ROM and strengthening exercises can be started.

### 3.8.4   Return to Sport

Patient may return to non-contact sport when the patient is free of symptoms and full return is possible when complete healing takes place, usually 8–10 weeks.

## 3.9   Burst Fracture

Burst fracture is a descriptive term for an injury to a vertebral body in which it is severely compressed. The usual cause is severe trauma in which a great force is applied to the spine vertically and causes the vertebral body to be compressed on all sides. This differs from a compression fracture, in which only the anterior part of the vertebral body is crushed. The patient usually relays a story of a jump or a fall in which he or she landed firmly on the feet, or perhaps directly on the pelvis. This type of fracture has more potential to cause neurological damage since the bony elements of the vertebral body are spread in all directions and the spinal cord, as well as the nerve roots, are more likely to be damaged. Also since all the margins of the vertebral body are compressed, this fracture causes the spine to be less stable compared with the compression fracture.

### 3.9.1   Clinical Presentation

The patient typically has pain at the level of the fractured vertebra. If there is neurological damage, then patients may offer complaints suggestive of radicular pain.

### 3.9.2   Diagnosis

Patients will generally be in severe pain, which may preclude any special testing, although a focused neurological exam will help determine the level and estimate the extent of injury. X-rays and CT scans will reveal loss of height of the vertebral body and extent of the damage sustained from the burst fracture, including the level of the fracture, extent of spinal canal compromise, and spinal angulation. MRI may be necessary to assess the amount of soft tissue trauma, bleeding, and ligament disruption.

### 3.9.3 Treatment

First it is essential to determine whether the burst fracture is stable. The burst fracture is considered to be stable if there is no neurological injury, spinal canal compromise is <50%, and the angulation is <20%. In the cases of stable fracture, the treatment is molded brace or a body cast worn for 8–12 weeks and has excellent prognosis. It is necessary to treat pain, especially during the first 3–4 weeks, when it is most acute. However it is necessary to keep a close follow-up since a fracture that was considered stable and treated with bracing may start to angulate while in the brace. If the fracture does not meet the criteria for a stable burst fracture described in the preceding, surgery will likely be necessary. After surgery or after 8–12 weeks of wearing the brace the patient should start physical therapy to strengthen the trunk and lower extremities.

### 3.9.4 Return to Sport

The patient should have full and pain free range of motion. The patient should be involved in a structured home exercise program to focus on core stabilization.

## References

1. Bellah RD, Summerville DA, Treves ST, Micheli LJ (1991) Low-back pain in adolescent athletes: detection of stress injury to the pars interarticularis with SPECT. Radiology 180:509–512
2. Bono CM (2004) Low-back pain in athletes. J Bone Joint Surg Am 86-A(2):382–396
3. Congeni J, McCulloch J, Swanson K (1997) Lumbar spondylolysis. A study of natural progression in athletes. Am J Sports Med 25:248–253
4. Cooke PM, Lutz GE (2000) Internal disc disruption and axial back pain in the athlete. Phys Med Rehabil Clin North Am 11(4):837–865
5. Duda M (1989) Golfers use exercise to get back in the swing. Phys Sportsmed 17:109–113
6. Fehlandt AF Jr, Micheli LJ (1993) Lumbar facet stress fracture in a ballet dancer. Spine 18:2537–2539
7. Fredericson M., Moore W, Biswal S (2007) Sacral stress fractures: magnetic resonance imaging not always definitive for early stage injuries: a report of 2 cases. Am. J Sports Med 35(5): 835–839
8. Gatt CJ Jr, Hosea TM, Palumbo RC, Zawadsky JP (1997) Impact loading of the lumbar spine during football blocking. Am J Sports Med 25:317–321
9. Guillodo Y, Botton E, Saraux A, Le Goff P (2000) Contralateral spondylolysis and fracture of the lumbar pedicle in an elite female gymnast: a case report. Spine 25:2541–2543
10. Hainline B (1995) Low back injury. Sports Med 14(1):241–265

11. Hickey GJ, Fricker PA, McDonald WA (1997) Injuries to elite rowers over a 10-yr period. Med Sci Sports Exerc 29:1567–1572
12. Hopkins TJ, White AA 3rd (1993) Rehabilitation of athletes following spine injury. Clin Sports Med 12:603–619
13. Ikata T, Miyake R, Katoh S, Morita T, Murase M (1996) Pathogenesis of sports-related spondylolisthesis in adolescents. Radiographic and magnetic resonance imaging study. Am J Sports Med 24:94–98
14. Jackson DW, Wiltse LL, Dingeman RD, Hayes M (1981) Stress reactions involving the pars interarticularis in young athletes. Am J Sports Med 9:304–312
15. Keene JS, Albert MJ, Springer SL, Drummond DS, Clancy WG Jr (1989) Back injuries in college athletes. J Spinal Disord 2:190–195
16. Kibler WB, Chandler TJ (2003) Range of motion in junior tennis players participating in an injury risk modification program. J Sci Med Sport 6:51–62
17. Kujala UM, Taimela S, Oksanen A, Salminen JJ (1997) Lumbar mobility and low back pain during adolescence. A longitudinal three-year follow-up study in athletes and controls. Am J Sports Med 25:363–368
18. McCarroll JR, Miller JM, Ritter MA (1986) Lumbar spondylolysis and spondylolisthesis in college football players. A prospective study. Am J Sports Med 14:404–406.
19. Nadler SF, Malanga GA, DePrince M, Stitik TP, Feinberg JH (2000) The relationship between lower extremity injury, low back pain, and hip muscle strength in male and female collegiate athletes. Clin J Sports Med 10:89–97
20. Nadler SF, Wu KD, Galski T, Feinberg JH (1998) Low back pain in college athletes. A prospective study correlating lower extremity overuse or acquired ligamentous laxity with low back pain. Spine 23:828–833
21. Ong A, Anderson J, Roche J (2003) A pilot study of the prevalence of lumbar disc degeneration in elite athletes with lower back pain at the Sydney 2000 Olympic Games. Br J Sports Med 37:263–266
22. Quinn S, Bird S (1996) Influence of saddle type upon the incidence of lower back pain in equestrian riders. Br J Sports Med 30:140–144
23. Salai M, Brosh T, Blankstein A, Oran A, Chechik A (1999) Effect of changing the saddle angle on the incidence of low back pain in recreational bicyclists. Br J Sports Med 33:398–400
24. Shah MK, Stewart GW (2002) Sacral stress fractures: an unusual cause of low back pain in an athlete. Spine 27:E104–108
25. Shelerud R (1998) Epidemiology of occupational low back pain. Occup Med 13:1–22
26. Soler T, Calderon C (2000) The prevalence of spondylolysis in the Spanish elite athlete. Am J Sports Med 28:57–62
27. Trainor TJ, Wiesel SW (2002) Epidemiology of back pain in the athlete. Clin Sports Med 21:93–103
28. Vad VB, Cano WG, Basrai D, Lutz GE, Bhat AL (2003) Role of radiofrequency denervation in lumbar zygapophyseal joint synovitis in baseball pitchers: a clinical experience. Pain Phys 6(3):307–312
29. Young JL, Press JM, Herring SA (1997) The disc at risk in athletes: perspectives on operative and nonoperative care. Med Sci Sports Exerc 29(7 Suppl):S222–232

# Chapter 9
# Hip Injuries

Necolle Morgado and Parag Sheth

## 1 Introduction

Hip pain occurs in many athletes. It can be a divided into acute injuries and chronic injuries. Acute injuries are usually the result of a traumatic event such as a collision, fall, or tackle and are seen in sports such as skiing, figure skating, gymnastics, rugby, and football. Acute injuries are also common in sports such as soccer, sprinting, hurdling, martial arts, and basketball, all of which require sudden acceleration or deceleration forces. Chronic overuse injuries are a result of repetitive motions at the hip joint and usually occur in running, golf, and ballet.

## 2 Anatomy

The hip joint is a multiaxial ball-and-socket synovial joint. It is a strong, stable joint that allows for a wide ROM. The hip relies on a combination of articular, ligamentous and muscular structures to achieve stability. Most of the hip joint's stability comes from the joint capsule rather than the surrounding musculature.

### 2.1 Bones

By the end of puberty, the mature hip is formed by the fusion of the ilium, ischium, and pubis. The hips form the connection between the lower limbs (femurs) and the vertebral column (sacrum). The two hip bones are joined anteriorly by the pubic symphysis and posteriorly articulate with the sacrum to form most of the bony pelvis.

### 2.2 Static Stabilizers

The static stabilizers of the hip include the acetabular labrum and the ligaments. The acetabular labrum extends beyond the bony rim of the acetabulum and increases the depth and overall surface area of the acetabulum. The acetabular labrum

J.E. Herrera and G. Cooper (eds.), *Essential Sports Medicine*, doi: 10.1007/978-1-59745-414-8, © Humana Press 2008 functions to hold the head of the femur in place so that a complete socket is formed. The primary ligaments of the hip are the iliofemoral ligament (Y ligament of Bigelow), pubofemoral, ischiofemoral, ligamentum orbicularis, and ligamentum teres. The ligaments form a capsule that contains the head and neck of the femur and stabilizes the hip by restraining extension, abduction, and internal rotation of the femur.

## 2.3  Dynamic Stabilizers

There are many muscles that cross the hip joint, including the rectus femoris and hamstrings, but the major dynamic stabilizers of the hip include the glutei (minimus, medius, and maximus), iliopsoas, iliacus, psoas major, adductors, iliotibial band with the tensor fasciae latae, and deep musculature (pectineus, piriformis, superior and inferior gemellus, and obturator internus and externus). These deep muscles of the hip are thought to be the "rotator cuff" muscles of the hip and have a role in fine-tuning hip motions.

## 2.4  Biomechanics

Like the shoulder, the ball-and-socket design makes the hip one of the most movable of all joints. However, the hip is more stable than the shoulder because unlike the shoulder, which has a mobile scapula, the head of the femur has adequate coverage and containment within the acetabulum.

The amount of acetabular coverage of the femoral head is one important element for proper hip biomechanics. The degree of femoral head coverage by the acetabulum is measured radiographically as the center-edge angle, or angle of Wiberg. The angle of Wiberg is obtained by drawing a horizontal line through the center of the femoral head and a line tangent to the superior and inferior acetabular rims. Normal is 30–40 degrees. Poor femoral head coverage by the acetabulum results in an abnormal orientation of the acetabulum and less than satisfactory load transfer.

There are two additional anatomical geometries of the femur and acetabulum that are important to providing an appropriate femoral head position within the capsule and maintaining joint stability and mobility: appropriate femoral head–neck offset and acetabular anteversion. Femoral head–neck offset is the distance between the most superior aspect of the femoral head and the femoral neck. This is obtained by drawing a line through the long axis of the femoral neck and drawing lines parallel to it to indicate the most superior aspect of the femoral head and femoral neck. The amount of offset from the femoral head to the femoral neck must be enough to allow full ROM without impinging on the acetabular labrum. Femoroacetabular impingement can result from a lack of offset from the femoral head to the femoral neck.

Normal anteversion of the acetabulum is also essential in maintaining a normal relationship with the femoral head and is critical in avoiding impingement. Acetabular anteversion represents the anterior direction of the acetabulum. Normal range of acetabular anteversion is 20 degrees.

Also important to hip stability is the femoral neck–shaft angle. The femoral neck is angled at 120–130 degrees relative to the femoral shaft. A decrease in neck–shaft angle is called coxa vara, and an increase is termed coxa valga. The primary hip flexor is the iliopsoas, which can achieve 120 degrees of flexion. The hip extensors include the gluteus maximus and hamstring muscles, which provide the hip with 30 degrees of extension. There are 45–50 degrees of abduction in the hip joint, and the primary abductors are the gluteus medius and minimus muscles. The main adductors of the hip are the adductor longus, gracilis, pectineus, adductor brevis, and adductor magnus. There are approximately 20–30 degrees of adduction in the hip.

# 3   Acute Hip Injuries

## 3.1   Acetabular Labral Tears

An acetabular labral tear commonly occurs with hyperextension and external rotation of the femur. There is a high incidence of acetabular labral tears in athletes who participate in sports that require frequent external rotation at the hip joint, such as soccer, hockey, golf, and ballet. Some tears have also been attributed to running and sprinting. Major trauma, such as hip dislocation, can also result in acetabular tears.

### 3.1.1   Clinical Presentation

Athletes commonly complain of pain in the anterior hip or groin pain with motion. Less often the patient may complain of pain deep in the posterior buttocks. The patient can also report of locking, clicking, or giving way at the hip. These symptoms usually have a gradual onset unless related to trauma.

### 3.1.2   Diagnosis

On physical exam, there will be significant pain with hip flexion, medial rotation, and adduction. Depending on the severity, an acetabular labral tear can also present with subluxation. If the diagnosis is not apparent on initial physical exam, then resisted straight leg raising test should be performed.

In the resisted straight-leg raise test, the patient lies supine. The examiner asks the patient to elevate the entire leg off the examining table while the knee is extended. The examiner then applies resistance to the leg; reproduction of pain presents a positive test.

Diagnostic studies such as x-rays and MRIs may be useful for detecting and diagnosing labral pathology. Standard radiographs are typically normal, although the radiographs of some patients may show dysplasia, degenerative changes, or subtle bony abnormalities. Conventional MRI and MR arthrography are the most accurate in identifying labral tears. Contrast along the acetabular labral interface, with or without displacement of the labrum from the acetabulum, are some of the criteria used to define a labral tear.

Currently the gold standard for diagnosis of labral tears is direct observation of the labrum by arthroscopy.

### 3.1.2.1  Grading and Classification Based on Etiology and Morphology

- *Radial flap tear:* Most common, involves disruption of the free margin of the labrum with formation of a flap of labral tissue
- *Radial fibrillated tear:* Has the appearance of chronic degenerative change and is more commonly seen in patients with degenerated articular cartilage
- *Longitudinal peripheral tear:* Seen at the junction of the acetabular rim and the labrum
- *Mobile tear:* Unstable structure, associated with pain on motion and subluxation

### 3.1.3  Treatment

Conservative treatment includes NSAIDs, limited weight bearing, and physical therapy. Therapy should focus on instructing the patient to avoid pivoting motions, specifically hip rotation under load. Surgery can involve arthroscopic debridement of the labral tear or partial labrectomy (excision of the torn tissue), which remains the treatment of choice regardless of classification of tear.

### 3.1.4  Return to Play

Before an athlete with an acetabular tear returns to play, the athlete should have full painless passive and active ROM. Drills emphasizing speed are added to the training program and ROM is assessed at every training session. Any return of pain and/or stiffness should warrant a cutback in activity and change in exercise regimen and return to play schedule.

## 3.2  Groin Strain or Hip Adductor Strain

A groin strain is also known as a hip adductor strain. This is the most common cause of groin pain in athletes. This injury occurs secondary to resisted forceful abduction or adduction of the hip, such as a forced push-off (side-to-side) motion, during a sudden change of direction while running, and quick starts and stops. Factors such as weakness or tightness of the adductor muscles can predispose an athlete to a groin strain. This injury is commonly seen in soccer players as well as football, ice hockey, basketball, tennis, and baseball players.

### 3.2.1  Clinical Presentation

An athlete usually presents with pain with resisted adduction and sometimes pain with hip flexion.

### 3.2.2  Diagnosis

Physical exam usually reveals pain on palpation of the adductor muscle and pain on adduction against resistance. Pain can also be reproduced with passive abduction. A palpable defect may be appreciated.

Diagnostic studies such as radiographs of the hip focusing on the adductor tubercle are important to rule out an adductor avulsion fracture. MRI can be used to confirm muscle strain or partial or complete tendon tears. Ultrasound is useful for diagnosing muscle and tendon tears but not muscle strains.

### 3.2.3  Treatment

Initial treatment consists of RICE and NSAIDs, followed by physical therapy with the goal of restoring ROM and preventing atrophy. The patient should then progress to stretching and strengthening exercises as well as focus on improving flexibility and endurance.

Patients with chronic adductor strains who have failed to respond to conservative treatment should be considered for surgical tenotomy.

### 3.2.4  Return to Play

Return to sport may be allowed when the athlete has regained at least 70% of his or her strength and has pain-free full ROM. This may take 4–8 weeks for an acute strain and up to 6 months for a chronic strain.

## 3.3  Piriformis Syndrome

Piriformis syndrome can occur in athletes after forceful hip internal rotation. In severe cases, the sciatic nerve may be involved because the nerve goes through the muscle fibers of the piriformis in some individuals.

### 3.3.1   Clinical Presentation

Athletes complain of lateral buttock pain and/or pain in the proximal posterior thigh, posterior hip, and sacroiliac region. The pain is usually worse with standing and walking up the stairs.

### 3.3.2   Diagnosis

On physical exam there is pain with passive internal rotation, adduction, and flexion of the hip. There is also tenderness from the sacrum to the greater trochanter.

Diagnostic studies such as x-rays of the L/S spine and hip may be helpful to rule out other pathology.

### 3.3.3   Treatment

Initial treatment consists of ultrasound, NSAIDs, and stretching of the external rotator hip muscles. The goal is to reduce pain and spasm and recover full hip internal rotation. If these more conservative treatments fail, local corticosteroid injections can be used.

### 3.3.4   Return to Play

The athlete can return to play when he or she can demonstrate full pain-free ROM and strength of the affected side and can perform sport-specific activities without discomfort. The time it takes for return to play varies with each individual and the type of treatment the patient received. The longer an athlete waits to receive treatment, the longer it will take for the patient to return to play.

## 3.4   Hamstring Strain

Hamstring strain usually occurs as a result of poor flexibility, poor conditioning, inadequate warm-up, muscle imbalance, repetitive microtrauma, overuse, and exercise fatigue. Injuries usually occur during the eccentric phase of contraction. Hamstring strain is common in track athletes and gymnasts.

### 3.4.1   Grading and Classification

- *First degree:* Stretch injury
- *Second degree:* Partial tear
- *Third degree:* Complete rupture

### 3.4.2   Clinical Presentation

The athlete usually experiences pain after a forceful knee extension or hamstring contraction. He or she may also experience tenderness over the muscle origin or the belly of the muscle. In third degree strain there is an acute loss of muscular function.

### 3.4.3   Diagnosis

Physical exam reveals pain in the ischial region of the pelvis with resisted flexion of the knee or pain with flexion of the hip with the knee extended. A palpable defect may be present.

Diagnostic studies are generally not needed, but MRI is useful in distinguishing acute from chronic muscle strain. Acute muscle strain often affects the myotendinous junction and chronic injuries usually involve the tendon.

### 3.4.4   Treatment

Initial treatment consists of rest, ice, NSAIDs, compression, weight-bearing reduction if necessary, and gentle stretch. Once inflammation is reduced, strengthening exercises can be started.

### 3.4.5   Return to Play

The athlete may return to play when the affected hamstring has full ROM and at least 90% of the strength of the healthy hamstring. Before return to play can be considered it is also important that the athlete achieves normal flexibility and endurance.

## 3.5   Avulsion Injuries

Avulsion injuries are common in athletes, especially adolescents due to an inherent weakness of apophysis. Acute avulsion injuries occur as a result of extreme active contraction or sudden passive lengthening of a muscle. Avulsion fractures most commonly occur at the ischial tuberosity. Other common sites are the anterior superior iliac spine (ASIS), anterior inferior iliac spine (AIIS), the lesser and greater trochanter as well as the pubic bone.

The ischial tuberosity is the origin of the hamstrings tendon and is the site of a hamstring avulsion after forceful hamstring contraction with the knee in extension and hip in flexion. These injuries are commonly seen in sports involving sprinting and hurdling.

ASIS avulsion fractures are caused by sudden contraction of the sartorius muscle when the hip is extended and the knee flexed. This injury is common in sports requiring jumping and in sprinters after forceful hip extension. AIIS avulsion injuries are caused by strong rectus femoris contractions and occur after forceful kicking in sports such as soccer.

### 3.5.1 Clinical Presentation

Athletes with an ischial tuberosity avulsion may present with sudden onset of severe pain and immediate loss of function. They may complain of buttock pain, difficulty sitting, altered gait, or even an inability to ambulate. Patients with an ASIS avulsion injury may also complain of paresthesias involving the anterolateral thigh and pain when they flex the hip (sitting) because of secondary meralgia paresthesias. Athletes with an AIIS avulsion injury present with acute onset of pain over the AIIS or groin pain.

### 3.5.2 Diagnosis

The physical exam in an athlete with ischial tuberosity avulsion will reveal pain and tenderness over the ischial tuberosity. Pain can be reproduced with hip flexion with the knee extended. Physical exam of a patient with an ASIS avulsion will reveal pain and localized tenderness and/or swelling with palpation over the ASIS. Hip flexion and abduction provokes symptoms. Patients with AIIS avulsion will reveal pain on contraction of quadriceps as well as pain with hip extension or hip flexion. There may also be localized swelling in the region of AIIS.

If a diagnosis is not made after performing the basic physical exam, the straight leg raising test can be done. This test will be positive (reproduction of the patient's pain) in patients with ischial tuberosity avulsion.

Diagnostic studies such as x-ray of hip with frog leg view and MRI will reveal avulsion (displacement of the involved area, i.e., ASIS, AIIS, ischial tuberosity).

### 3.5.3 Treatment

For ischial, ASIS, and AIIS avulsion injuries the initial treatment is bed rest with the hip and knee flexed and application of ice to the affected area. Weight-bearing and ambulation as tolerated follow this. Resistive exercises can be started once the athlete achieves a full ROM. Stretching, functional strengthening, and proprioceptive activities are then started. Athletes with ASIS avulsions may need splinting of the knee in flexion to reduce tension on the avulsion segment.

Surgery is required for a displaced apophysis. Displacement of the avulsed fragment >2 cm may require surgical fixation.

### 3.5.4   Return to Play

Athletes that suffered an ASIS avulsion injury can usually return to full level of activity within 5–6 weeks, as compared with athletes with an ischial tuberosity/ hamstring avulsion injury, who require a longer recovery time.

## 3.6   Stress Fractures of the Femoral Neck

Stress fractures are caused by repetitive overload and overuse. Stress fractures are classified into two types based on etiology: insufficiency fractures and fatigue fractures. Insufficiency fractures are most commonly seen in the elderly population with osteoporosis and other underlying bone diseases and are defined as fractures of abnormal bone subjected to normal forces.

Fatigue fractures are most often seen in young athletes, especially those involved in running and jumping, and are seen in endurance athletes such as military recruits. These are fractures that occur when normal bone is subjected to abnormal forces. Risk factors for fatigue stress fractures are female gender and low femoral bone mineral density scores. Fatigue fractures are the focus of this section.

### 3.6.1   Clinical Presentation

The athletes usually present with an antalgic gait and report progressive activity-related pain in the groin or anterior thigh that is alleviated with rest. The pain can become constant if the athlete continues the activity. Patients usually report a history of participating in a new activity that involves strenuous, repetitive movements.

### 3.6.2   Diagnosis

On physical exam, there may be a focal area of increased tenderness, erythema, warmth, and swelling. A region of periosteal thickening may be palpable. Physical exam reveals pain at extreme ranges of external and internal rotation, and there may also be painful limitation of internal rotation of the hip. Special tests, such as the single-leg hop test, reproduces symptoms.

Diagnostic studies such as radiographs, bone scintigraphy, and MRI are useful in detecting stress fractures. X-rays of the hip may be normal initially; when changes are present they normally lag behind the onset of symptoms by 2–4 weeks and may show a radiolucent line or periosteal thickening. If the x-rays are negative, bone scan or MRI should be performed. Bone scans may be positive 2–8 days after onset of symptoms and are more sensitive and specific when compared with plain films. The combination of radiographs and bone scan allows for a correct diagnosis in 90% of cases. MRI is more accurate, specific, and sensitive when compared with bone scintigraphy. MRI has the advantage of greater localization and grading of injury severity and in differentiating stress fracture from other bone and soft tissue conditions such as avascular necrosis.

### 3.6.3 Classification

Fatigue fractures of the femoral neck are further classified based on the mechanism of injury.

Compression-type fractures are more common and occur along the inferior femoral neck. This fracture is stable and has a good prognosis for healing.

Transverse/distraction-type fractures develop across the superior surface of the femur and continue across to the femoral neck. This fracture has a high risk of displacement and athletes with this injury should always be referred to an orthopedic surgeon for management.

### 3.6.4 Treatment

Compression-type fractures are more stable and therefore treated with bed rest. Once the patient has little to no pain at rest he or she can progress to non-weight bearing with crutches with frequent repeat radiographs. When radiographs demonstrate evidence of complete healing, progressive weight bearing and activity are permitted.

Recurrence of pain warrants rest for 2–3 days, then resumption of activity at the last level tolerated. Surgery with internal fixation may be indicated if the fracture progresses.

Transverse-type fractures require surgery with open reduction and internal fixation because of the high risk of progression to complete fracture, displacement, and avascular necrosis. Patient should be non-weight bearing for 6 weeks followed by 6 weeks of partial weight bearing. A displaced fracture is an orthopedic emergency requiring immediate surgical reduction and fixation.

### 3.6.5 Return to Play

With compression type fractures return to play occurs in 2–3 months.

## 4 Chronic Hip Injuries

### 4.1 Osteitis Pubis

Osteitis pubis is an inflammatory condition of the joint of the pubic rami. It is characterized by pain at the pubic symphysis and joint disruption. It occurs as a result of increased stress placed on the joint from the traction of the pelvic musculature or from repetitive stress causing increased shearing forces on the pubic symphysis. This injury is common in soccer players and distance runners.

### 4.1.1  Clinical Presentation

The athlete may report a gradual increase in pain in the lower abdomen and medial thigh with exercise. The pain will slowly progress in severity if activities are not stopped. Athletes may complain of adductor pain, pain around the pubic symphysis, lower abdominal pain, and hip pain. Athletes may complain of "popping" in the pubic region with normal ambulation. Pain referred to the scrotum can occur but is less common.

### 4.1.2  Diagnosis

On physical exam there may be tenderness over the pubic symphysis. If the distal symphysis is involved, then pain is exacerbated by active adduction. If the proximal portion is involved, then the pain is provoked by sit-ups. A special test that can be performed to confirm diagnosis is having the patient hop on one leg and if the patient complains of pain in the groin or pubic region this is a positive test.

Plain radiographs may be normal in early or mild disease. As the disease progresses the plain radiographs may demonstrate widening of the pubic symphysis, periarticular sclerosis, or an irregular contour of the articular surfaces. Bone scans may show increased uptake in the area of the pubic symphysis. MRI can show marrow edema in the pubic bones.

### 4.1.3  Treatment

The first line of treatment is usually rest and NSAIDs, followed by physical therapy. Therapy should focus on ROM exercises of the hip as well as adductor stretching and strengthening exercises. Pain-free exercise should be continued in order to maintain physical fitness, and activities that exacerbate pain should be avoided.

Corticosteroid injections are controversial but have been shown to be helpful in certain patients, such as athletes with acute osteitis (<2 weeks duration). Surgery for arthrodesis may be required in severe cases.

### 4.1.4  Return to Play

If possible, return to play occurs once the patient is completely pain-free. Patients may be allowed to return to play prior to being pain-free since the disease is self-limited and resolves within 6–12 months.

## 4.2   Greater Trochanter Bursitis

Bursitis is defined as inflammation of the bursa over the greater trochanter and deep to the gluteus minimus, tensor fasciae latae, and gluteus medius, and occurs from excessive rubbing and friction. It can also develop after a direct blow causing hematoma formation.

Trochanteric bursitis is caused by the repetitive use of muscles that insert into the greater trochanter. This repetitive use results in degenerative changes of the surrounding tendons, soft tissues, and muscles. Trochanteric bursitis is associated with obesity, osteoarthritis, leg length discrepancy, overuse, direct trauma, and herniated lumbar disc, all of which cause muscle imbalance and reduced flexibility.

### 4.2.1   Clinical Presentation

Athlete experience intermittent, achy pain over the lateral aspect of the hip and complain of the inability to lie on the affected side secondary to pain. Patients may also complain of pain that radiates from hip to groin or into the lateral thigh. Symptoms are also exacerbated by prolonged standing, stair climbing, or running. They may also complain of hip snapping.

### 4.2.2   Diagnosis

On physical exam, a snap may be palpable over the greater trochanter and there may be a leg length discrepancy. The patients will have pain with palpation of the greater trochanter and pain with movement, especially external rotation and abduction and by resisted abduction. If diagnosis is not made on physical exam a special test that can be performed is the Patrick's (FABER) test. The Patrick's test is performed by placing the hip in flexion, abduction, and external rotation. This test will be positive in patients with greater trochanter bursitis.

Diagnostic studies are performed to rule out femoral neck stress fractures. Plain films of the hip may reveal calcifications in the region of the greater trochanter in up to 40% of patients. MRI may show increased signal around the greater trochanter.

### 4.2.3   Treatment

Bed rest, ice, NSAIDs, and physical therapy focusing on iliotibial band stretching and strengthening of the hip adductor muscles are the initial treatments. In severe cases, a cane may be needed for additional support and stability while ambulating. Local glucocorticoid anesthetic injections are also helpful to alleviate pain in resistant patients.

### 4.2.4 Return to Play

The athlete can return to play once he or she has developed adequate flexibility and is pain-free.

## 4.3 Iliopsoas Bursitis

Iliopsoas bursitis is caused by overuse and friction as the tendon slides over the iliopectineal eminence of the pubis. It is common in sports that require extensive use of hip flexors such as soccer, ballet, jumping, hurdling, and uphill running.

### 4.3.1 Clinical Presentation

The athlete may complain of hip snapping, as well as anterior hip or deep groin pain. Depending on the severity of the bursitis, the athlete may have a limp.

### 4.3.2 Diagnosis

On physical exam, hip extension (stretching of the iliopsoas) exacerbates symptoms. There may be pain on deep palpation of the femoral triangle where the musculotendinous junction of the iliopsoas can be palpated. Pain may also be reproduced when the patient raises the heel off the table at approximately 15 degrees while supine, which emphasizes the iliopsoas since it is the only active hip flexor in this position.

MRI is the diagnostic study of choice to identify iliopsoas bursitis. MRI may reveal a collection of fluid adjacent to the muscle and will rule out underlying bony pathology.

### 4.3.3 Treatment

Treatment consists of rest, ice, NSAIDs, and stretching of rotators and flexors of the hip followed by strengthening exercises with gradual return to sport. Corticosteroid injections can be helpful if conservative methods fail. Surgery is needed in refractory cases.

### 4.3.4 Return to Play

The athlete can return to play once he or she is pain-free and has achieved sufficient flexibility as well as adequate hip flexor strength.

## 4.4 Sports Hernias

Sports hernias are caused by weakening of the posterior inguinal wall, resulting in a direct or indirect hernia.

### 4.4.1 Clinical Presentation

Athletes can complain of a chronic, gradually worsening, diffuse, deep groin pain. Patients may also complain of increased pain with activities that increase intra-abdominal pressure (Valsalva). Male patients can complain of testicular pain.

### 4.4.2 Diagnosis

On physical exam there will be no clinically detectable inguinal hernia because only the posterior abdominal wall is involved in a sports hernia. Exam may reveal pain along the inguinal ligament and/or rectus muscles. If the physical exam is inconclusive, a test that can support this diagnosis is pain with the Valsalva maneuver.

Diagnostic studies such as radiographs, bone scans, and MRI are not useful in diagnosing sports hernia but may help exclude other causes of groin and hip pain. Ultrasound has been found to be useful for evaluating posterior abdominal wall deformities characteristic of sports hernias.

### 4.4.3 Treatment

Conservative treatment is rarely successful and if symptoms persist, the patient should undergo surgical exploration and repair, which has been reported to have a 90% success rate.

## 4.5 Snapping Hip Syndrome

Snapping hip is an audible click or snapping sensation that occurs around the hip. It may be painless or painful. Snapping hip syndrome is common in ballet dancers, gymnasts, basketball players, and track and field athletes.

### 4.5.1 Classification

1. *External/lateral:* More common; occurs when iliotibial band, tensor muscle of fascia lata, gluteus medius, or gluteus maximus muscle tendon rides back and forth across the greater trochanter. This may also cause bursitis to develop.

2. *Interior/medial/anterior:* Causes include iliopsoas tendon passing over iliopectineal eminence, acetabular labral tears, subluxation of the hip, and loose bodies.

The most common cause of a snapping hip is the iliotibial band sliding over the greater trochanter.

### 4.5.2  Clinical Presentation

The athlete may complain of a snapping sensation felt around the hip with movement that has been present for several months or years. The location may be described as deep in the groin or lateral in the hip. Some may complain of pain when snapping is felt, which is usually described as dull or aching in nature.

### 4.5.3  Diagnosis

On physical exam the patient with external snapping hip syndrome may have pain or tenderness over the lateral aspect of the gluteus maximus, proximal iliotibial band, or trochanteric bursa. This patient may also have a leg length discrepancy, iliotibial band tightness on the affected side, and weakness of the external rotators and hip abductors. Patients with internal snapping hip syndrome may demonstrate an anterior pelvic tilt due to a tight iliopsoas tendon and snapping may be reproduced with extension of the flexed, abducted, and externally rotated hip.

If diagnosis is not apparent on basic physical exam, a test that can be performed to better identify external snapping hip syndrome consists of passive internal and external rotation of the hip with the patient in the side-lying position, which will reproduce the patient's symptoms. In contrast, a patient with internal snapping hip syndrome will have reproduction of symptoms with extension of the affected leg from a flexed, abducted, and externally rotated position.

Diagnostic studies such as plain films are not necessary if the diagnosis based on history and physical is definitive, especially since the majority of plain films are within normal limits. Ultrasound can be a useful diagnostic test because it may demonstrate changes in anatomy and provide the ability to directly visualize the iliopsoas tendon. MRI also can be used to better visualize the hip anatomy and may demonstrate significant findings in patients with snapping hip syndrome. For example, in a patient with involvement of the iliotibial band, the T2-weighted images on MRI may show fluid in the trochanteric bursa. In cases in which the iliopsoas tendon is involved, the T2-weighted images may demonstrate the affected tendon to be thicker relative to the unaffected side. There may also be fluid in or around the iliopsoas bursa.

### 4.5.4  Treatment

Treatment consists of NSAIDs, rest, activity modification, and physical therapy. Patients are instructed to eliminate repetitive motion activities such as running until they are asymptomatic. Therapy initially focuses on the use of modalities such as ice, electrical stimulation, and ultrasound, and then progresses to strengthening and stretching exercises as tolerated. Crutches can be used in severe cases. Corticosteroid injection may be useful for patients who continue to have pain and have failed other treatments.

In addition, hip arthroscopy may be considered to rule out other pathology such as a labral tear. Surgery may be an option for patients who continue to suffer from persistent pain and have failed other conservative treatments, although surgery is rarely necessary. The surgical interventions that are used for external snapping hip syndrome include various resections of the iliotibial band with excision of the trochanteric bursa and z-plasty of the iliotibial band resulting in lengthening of the tendon. Surgery for internal snapping hip syndrome consists of lengthening or complete release of the iliopsoas tendon and/or resection of the bony prominence of the lesser trochanter.

### 4.5.5 Return to Play

It is safe for the athlete to return to play once he or she is pain-free and able to perform sports-specific activities. Prior to return to play the patient also should be able to demonstrate full strength and flexibility of the involved lower extremity. Patients are encouraged to return to activities as tolerated.

## References

1. Akermark C, Johansson C (1992) Tenotomy of the adductor longus tendon in the treatment of chronic pain in athletes. Am J Sports Med 20:640–643
2. Anderson K, Strickland SM, Warren R (2001) Hip and groin injuries in athletes. Am J Sports Med 29:521–533
3. Armfield DR, Hyun-Min Kim D, Towers JD, Bradley JP, Robertson DD (2006) Sports-related muscle injury in the lower extremity. Clin Sports Med 25(4)
4. Brignall CG, Stainsby GD (1991) The snapping hip. Treatment by Z-plasty. J Bone Joint Surgery Br 73(2):253–254
5. Browning KH (2001) Hip and pelvis injuries in runners. Phys Sports Med 29:6
6. Cuccurullo SJ (2004) Hip disorders. Phys Med Rehabil Board Rev 208
7. Egol KA, Koval KJ, Kummer F (1998) Stress fractures of the femoral neck. Clin Orthop 348(Mar):72–78
8. Estwanik JJ, Sloane B, Rosenberg MA (1990) Groin strain and other possible causes of groin pain. Sports Med 18:59–65
9. Hase T, Ueo T (1999) Acetabular labral tear: arthroscopic diagnosis and treatment. Arthroscopy 15:138–141
10. Hoelmich P (1997) Adductor-related groin pain in athletes. Sports Med Arthrosc Rev 5:285–291
11. Holt MA, Keene JS, Graf BK, Helwig DC (1995) Treatment of osteitis pubis in athletes. Results of corticosteroid injections. Am J Sports Med 23:601
12. Jacobson T, Allen WC (1990) Surgical correction of the snapping iliopsoas tendon. Am J Sports Med 18(5):470–474

13. Johnston CA, Wiley JP, Lindsay DM, Wiseman DA (1998) Iliopsoas bursitis and tendinitis. Sports Med 25:271–283
14. Karlsson J, Jerre R (1997) The use of radiography, magnetic resonance, and ultrasound in the diagnosis of hip, pelvis, and groin injuries. Sports Med Arthroscop Rev 5:268–273
15. Keskula DR, Tamburello M (1992) Conservative management of piriformis syndrome. J Athletic Train 27(2):102, 104, 106–107
16. Lewis CL, Sahrmann SA (2006) Acetabular labral tears. J Amer Phys Ther Assoc 86:110–121
17. Lynch SA, Renstrom PA (1999) Groin injuries in sport: treatment strategies. Sports Med 28:137–144
18. Mason JB (2001) Acetabular labral tears in the athlete. Clin Sports Med 20:779–790
19. Morelli V, Smith V (2001) Groin injuries in athletes. Am Fam Phys 64:9
20. Nicholas SJ, Tyler TF (2002) Adductor muscle strain in sport. Sports Med 32(5)339–344
21. Overdeck KH, Palmer WE (2004) Imaging of hip and groin injuries in athletes. Semin Musculo Radiol 8:42–50
22. Pavlov H, Nelson TL, Warren RF (1982) Stress fractures of the pubic ramus: a report of twelve cases. J Bone Joint Surg (Am) 64(7):1020–1025
23. Schaberg JE, Harper MC, Allen WC (1984) The snapping hip syndrome. Am J Sports Med 12(5):361–365
24. Shbeeb MI, Matteson EL (1996) Trochanteric bursitis (greater trochanter pain syndrome). Mayo Clinic Proc 71 (6):565–569
25. Sorry MR, Schenker ML, Martin HD, Hogoboom D, Philippon MJ (2006) Neuromuscular hip biomechanics and pathology in the athlete. Clin Sports Med 25:180,189
26. Steiner C, Staubs C, Ganon M, Buhlinger C (1987) Piriformis syndrome: pathogenesis, diagnosis and treatment. J Am Osteopath Assoc 87(4):318–323

# Chapter 10
# Knee Injuries

Marc Effron and Gregory E. Lutz

## 1 Introduction

Injuries to the knee are among the most common sports-related injuries. Approximately one third of patients presenting to outpatient sports clinics have sustained knee injuries. Injuries to the knee can be seen in both contact and non-contact sports. Acute and chronic overuse injuries are common. Acute injuries can occur in sports such as football, basketball, and soccer that require frequent acceleration, deceleration, pivoting, and jumping. Overuse injuries usually result from poor biomechanics in sports such as marathon running and cycling.

## 2 Anatomy

### 2.1 Introduction

The knee joint is a modified hinge joint that allows the leg to flex and extend. It is the largest joint in the body in terms of its volume and surface area of articular cartilage. The knee joint also has one of the most complex articulations, allowing for the greatest susceptibility to injury and age-related degeneration.

### 2.2 Biomechanics

The knee joint consists of three compartments that all share a common synovial cavity. The medial tibiofemoral and lateral tibiofemoral compartments are involved in weight-bearing activities. The patellofemoral compartment contains the patella, which functions to increase the mechanical advantage of the quadriceps muscles. The fibular head lies within the capsule of the knee but is not usually involved in weight-bearing activities.

The knee typically permits approximately 135 degrees of flexion and 0 to −10 degrees of extension. ROM is limited in internal and external rotation. The average

J.E. Herrera and G. Cooper (eds.), *Essential Sports Medicine*,
doi: 10.1007/978-1-59745-414-8, © Humana Press 2008

knee permits about 10 degrees of internal rotation and 10 degrees of external rotation.

Studies have shown that the tibiofemoral shear force (tibial force on femur) is posterior at the tibiofemoral joint during muscle activity. The magnitude of the posterior shear force increases with knee flexion during closed kinetic chain exercise (foot is fixed and cannot move). During open kinetic chain exercise (foot is free to move) the resultant shear forces are maximal. This is an important consideration when deciding an appropriate rehabilitation program for the patient with an injured knee.

## 2.3   Bones

The knee is comprised of four bones. The femur, tibia, fibula, and patella are held together by strong ligaments, muscles, and a joint capsule. All four bones are lined with articular cartilage on their surfaces, which function to provide shock absorption.

The femur articulates with the tibia. The primary motion is flexion and extension. Axial rotation occurs when the knee is flexed. The bony anatomy of the tibia provides added stability during extension. The patella is a sesamoid bone embedded within the extensor muscle-tendon unit. The fibula articulates with the tibia and provides added stability.

## 2.4   Ligaments

The ligaments provide stability to the knee joint. The capsular ligaments consist of the medial collateral ligament, lateral collateral ligament, oblique popliteal ligament, and the arcuate popliteal ligament. The medial (tibial) collateral ligament connects the femur and the tibia on the medial side of the knee. It has an attachment directly to the medial meniscus. The lateral (fibular) collateral ligament connects the femur and the tibia on the lateral side of the knee. The oblique popliteal ligament and the arcuate popliteal ligament provide primarily posterior and lateral stability to the knee joint. The arcuate ligament has an attachment to the posterior horn of the lateral meniscus.

Internal stability of the knee is afforded by the crisscrossing of the anterior cruciate ligament and the posterior cruciate ligament. The anterior cruciate ligament functions primarily to restrain anterior tibial subluxation, whereas the posterior cruciate ligament helps restrain posterior tibial subluxation.

## 2.5   Menisci

The menisci provide shock absorption and enhance stability of the knee joint. There are two menisci located between the femoral and tibial articular surfaces. The medial and lateral menisci are biconcave, crescent-shaped, fibrocartilaginous discs. Their

blood supply originates from the periphery, thus the inner two thirds is not well vascularized. The menisci are attached to the joint plateau by small coronary ligaments.

## 2.6   Bursae

There are multiple bursae within the knee joint which function to reduce friction.
The four anterior bursae, three lateral bursae, three medial bursae, and two posterior
bursae all provide smooth motion during exercise.

## 2.7   Muscles

Several muscles encase the knee joint, providing motion and enhancing stability. The quadriceps muscle includes the rectus femoris, vastus lateralis, vastus
intermedius, and vastus medialis muscles. All four quads surround the patella
and join with the infrapatellar tendon to provide extension. The hamstrings,
which consist of the semimembranosus, semitendinosus, and biceps femoris,
are the principal flexors of the knee joint. The gastrocnemius facilitates flexion
and provides posterior stability. The gracilis and sartorius provide medial
rotation/flexion and medial stability. The popliteus and iliotibial band enhance
lateral stability.

# 3   Ligamentous Injuries

## 3.1   Anterior Cruciate Ligament

Anterior cruciate ligament (ACL) injuries are common in sports. The incidence of
ACL injury is greater in athletes who participate in contact sports such as football
or rugby. The mechanism of injury is usually hyperextension, deceleration, or cutting. Frequently, the ACL is injured in combination with other structures, such as
the medial collateral ligament and medial meniscus ("terrible triad"). In non-contact
sports such as skiing, the ACL is prone to injury when there is a force that drives
the tibia anteriorly while the knee is flexed at 90 degrees.

### 3.1.1   Clinical Presentation

Patients may admit to an audible "pop" that occurs while cutting or landing from a
jump. Early swelling may develop coinciding with severe knee pain. The patient
may be unable to fully extend the knee secondary to pain and swelling. Some
patients report a sensation of the knee "giving way" because of instability.

### 3.1.2 Diagnosis

On physical exam, the knee should be evaluated by inspection, assessing ROM, palpation, and testing for ligamentous laxity. Examine for an effusion. Tenderness is variable. There can be findings to suggest functional instability. Special tests are useful for establishing a diagnosis. The Lachman test (Fig. 10.1) is probably more sensitive for ACL dysfunction than the anterior drawer test.

- *Lachman test:* Have the patient lie supine with the knee flexed at 20–30 degrees. Attempt anterior translation by stabilizing the femur with one hand and apply an anterior stress to the proximal tibia with the other hand. A positive test occurs when there is excessive anterior translation with no distinct endpoint.
- *Anterior drawer test:* Have the patient lie supine with the knee flexed at 90 degrees. Sit gently on the patient's foot and grasp the patient's proximal tibia attempting forward translation. A positive test occurs when the tibia slides from under the femur with no distinct endpoint. Variations of this test include positioning the foot and leg in external and internal rotation while attempting forward translation. This maneuver helps assess the integrity of the posterome-dial and posterolateral joint capsule, respectively.
- *Pivot shift test:* Have the patient lie supine with the knee extended and the foot and leg internally rotated. Flex the knee to 20–30 degrees while applying a val-gus stress. The test is positive if the patient feels a sudden shift of the tibia anteriorly.

Diagnostic studies are useful for establishing a diagnosis. Anteroposterior and lateral radiographs are usually negative but may reveal an associated avulsion fracture. MRI is highly sensitive and specific, and should be considered in difficult

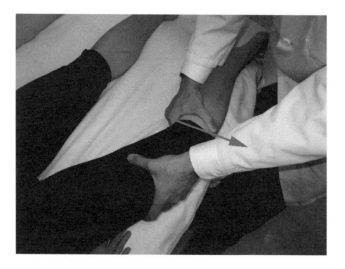

**Fig. 10.1** Lachman test

cases. Arthroscopy is the gold standard and useful for establishing associated intra-articular injuries.

ACL injuries are graded I–III. A grade I tear is a mild injury that causes microscopic tears in the ACL and does not affect overall weight-bearing. A grade II tear is a moderate injury in which the ACL is partially torn, causing some knee instability. A grade III tear is a severe injury in which the ACL is completely torn with resultant instability during weight-bearing.

### 3.1.3 Treatment

Initial treatment includes RICE, NSAIDs, and analgesics for pain control. Encourage partial weight-bearing with crutches while the patient is undergoing an evaluation. A limited motion brace may be used. If there is a significant effusion, a diagnostic or therapeutic aspiration may be considered. Patients should be referred for physical therapy.

A spectrum of physical therapy programs exist for the rehabilitation of the patient with an ACL injury. Research has shown that closed kinetic chain exercise is the preferred treatment since these maneuvers produce less shear forces at the tibiofemoral joint. It is the authors' opinion that the early stages of a comprehensive rehabilitation program should focus on protected mobilization and closed kinetic chain strengthening. Later stages should encompass neuromuscular-proprioceptive training and sports-specific agility training to redevelop the reaction time necessary for return to athletic competition.

Grades I and II injuries are usually managed conservatively with bracing and physical therapy. A grade III injury usually has a poor outcome with conservative care and thus requires a surgical consultation. Recurrent functional instability also necessitates a surgical consultation.

### 3.1.4 Return to Play

For grades I and II tears, athletes may return to play once quadriceps strength has been restored to 80% of the contralateral leg. For surgically treated ACL sprains, return to play can take up to 6–9 months.

## 3.2 Posterior Cruciate Ligament

Posterior cruciate ligament (PCL) injuries are less common than ACL injuries. This is a consequence of the PCL being much stronger and broader than the ACL. Injury to the PCL usually occurs when there is a blow to the front of the tibia while the knee is flexed. Injury may also occur following a rotational or valgus/varus stress with the knee in full extension or hyperextension. PCL injuries may occur in conjunction with other ligamentous injuries. Injuries to the PCL occur most often in contact sports such as football or rugby.

### 3.2.1 Clinical Presentation

Patients usually complain of minimal or no pain. Many are asymptomatic and can bear weight without significant discomfort. There can be associated swelling, although the overall extent is usually less than is seen in ACL injuries. Some patients report an audible "pop" following the traumatic event or a sensation of instability when walking. Patients may be unable to fully extend the leg.

### 3.2.2 Diagnosis

On physical exam, popliteal tenderness may be seen acutely. An effusion is sometimes noted. Abduction or adduction stress in full extension may elicit a positive test in cases of valgus or varus trauma. Special tests are useful for establishing a diagnosis.

- *Posterior drawer test:* Have the patient lie supine with the knee flexed at 90 degrees. Sit gently on the patient's foot and grasp the patient's proximal tibia attempting to push the tibia posteriorly (Fig. 10.2). A positive test occurs when there is excessive posterior translation with no distinct endpoint. A grade I injury is indicated when there is 0–5 mm of displacement and side-to-side asymmetry. A grade II injury or partial tear is suspected when there is 5–10 mm of displacement. A grade III injury or complete tear is indicated when there is >10 mm of displacement.

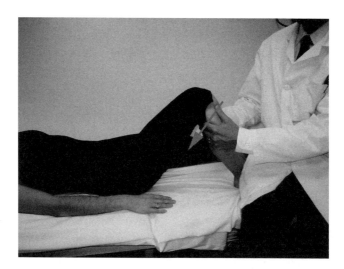

**Fig. 10.2** Posterior drawer test

- *Posterior sag test:* Also called the gravity test. Have the patient lie supine with both knees flexed at 90 degrees and feet flat on the table. Observe from the lateral side for posterior tibial displacement while comparing both legs. Note that a false-negative may occur with quadriceps spasm.

Diagnostic studies can be helpful for establishing a diagnosis. Anteroposterior and lateral radiographs are usually negative but may reveal an associated avulsion fracture. MRI should be considered in difficult cases.

### 3.2.3   Treatment

Initial treatment includes RICE, NSAIDs, and analgesics as needed for pain control. Grades I and II are usually managed conservatively with bracing and physical therapy. These patients can weight bear as tolerated but may require axillary crutches for comfort.

The rehabilitation program should begin with protected mobilization and closed kinetic chain strengthening. Later stages should include neuromuscular-proprioceptive training and sports-specific agility training to redevelop the reaction time necessary for return to play. Patients with a grade III injury or recurrent instability necessitate a surgical consultation. An isolated grade III tear can be managed conservatively with a long leg brace and crutches.

### 3.2.4   Return to Play

For grades I, II, and non-surgically treated grade III tears, patient may return to play once quadriceps strength has been regained. For surgically treated PCL sprains, return to play can take up to 9–12 months depending on compliance with physical therapy.

## 3.3   *Medial Collateral Ligament*

Medial collateral ligament (MCL) injuries are the most common among the ligamentous injuries. Injuries to the MCL result from a force directed to the lateral aspect of the knee. MCL injuries are common in contact sports such as football during a block against the lateral knee. Injuries to the MCL may also occur in non-contact sports such as skiing or swimming. Any sudden change in momentum or sustained valgus force at the knee can damage the MCL. Severe injury may also involve detachment of the medial meniscus or ACL.

### 3.3.1   Clinical Presentation

Patients present with medial knee pain after sustaining a lateral blow to the knee. Occasionally, patients may experience an audible "pop." The knee may stiffen within several hours. Grade III tears can still permit weight-bearing and adequate mobility once the acute pain resolves.

### 3.3.2  Diagnosis

On physical exam, tenderness is variable. Medial soft tissue swelling or ecchymosis may occur. Tests of medial instability are usually positive. Valgus stress should be performed at 30 degrees of flexion in order to grade the degree of MCL injury. In grade I injury, there is pain but no laxity with valgus stress indicating only microscopic damage. In grade II injury or partial tear, there is marked abduction of the leg with 5–10 mm of joint space opening, but a distinct endpoint is reached. In grade III injury or complete tear, there is >10 mm of joint space opening with no distinct endpoint reached.

Diagnostic studies can be useful in establishing a diagnosis. Routine radiographs are usually negative but may help rule out fractures of the distal femur, tibial plateau, or patella. MRI has high sensitivity and specificity for detecting MCL tears. MRI should be considered in patients who may have associated injuries to the ACL, PCL, or menisci.

### 3.3.3  Treatment

Initial treatment includes RICE, NSAIDs, and analgesics as needed. Grades I and II are managed with bracing and physical therapy. Crutches are used until weight-bearing is comfortable. The rehabilitation program should focus on stability and strengthening using closed kinetic chain exercises. A surgical consultation should be obtained for a grade III injury; however, most grade III tears are managed conservatively with functional bracing to prevent excessive valgus stress. Other complicated cases such as those involving associated ACL tears or avulsion fractures necessitate a surgical consultation.

### 3.3.4  Return to Play

Athletes are permitted to return to play when sport-specific function is pain-free and strength has returned to 90% of the uninjured leg. Patients with grades I and II sprains are often allowed to return to sports within 2–3 weeks. Grade III injuries usually require 6 or more weeks before return to play.

## 3.4  Lateral Collateral Ligament

Lateral collateral ligament (LCL) injuries are much less common than MCL injuries. This is due the contralateral leg protecting against a direct blow to the medial side of the knee. LCL injuries result from a varus force applied to the knee. LCL injuries are often seen in contact sports such as wrestling, soccer, or rugby. Occasionally, athletes may sustain an LCL injury during twisting as seen in tennis or racquetball.

### 3.4.1 Clinical Presentation

Patients present with lateral knee pain following a traumatic event. Assessing the mechanism of injury is important. Patients may describe a direct blow to the antero-medial aspect of the tibia. Additionally, they may describe a feeling of the knee "giving way" during pivoting or twisting activities.

### 3.4.2 Diagnosis

On physical exam, tenderness is variable. Lateral swelling may occur. Tests of lateral instability are usually positive. Varus stress should be performed at 30 degrees of flexion in order to grade the degree of LCL injury. In grade I injury, there is pain but no laxity, with varus stress indicating only microscopic damage. In grade II injury or partial tear, there is marked adduction of the leg with 5–10 mm of joint space opening, but a distinct endpoint is reached. In grade III injury or complete tear, there is >10 mm of joint space opening with no distinct end-point reached.

In acute injury, a positive posterolateral drawer test can be seen. In more chronic cases, a reverse pivot test and/or external rotation recurvatum test may be positive.

- *Reverse pivot test:* Have the patient lie supine with the knee flexed at 90 degrees and externally rotated. A positive test is seen when there is a palpable "clunk" during knee extension.
- *External rotation recurvatum test:* Have the patient lie supine. Lift both legs by the great toes. A positive test is seen with excessive recurvatum, external tibial rotation, and varus at the injured knee.

Diagnostic studies can be helpful in establishing a diagnosis. Routine radiographs are usually negative unless there is an associated avulsion fracture. MRI has high sensitivity and specificity for detecting LCL tears. MRI should be considered in difficult cases.

### 3.4.3 Treatment

Initial treatment includes RICE, NSAIDs, and analgesics as needed for pain control. Grades I and II are managed with bracing and physical therapy. Crutches should be prescribed for a reduction in weight-bearing. A return to full weight-bearing usually occurs over 4 weeks. The rehabilitation program should focus on stability and strengthening with closed kinetic chain exercises. A surgical consultation should be obtained for a grade III injury. Surgery is recommended for a grade III tear since this usually involves damage to the posterolateral capsular complex.

### 3.4.4   Return to Play

The timeframe for return to play depends on the severity of LCL injury and treatment received. After completing a physical therapy program, the athlete should demonstrate pain-free ROM with near-full strength.

## 4   Meniscal Injuries

### 4.1   *Medial and Lateral Meniscus*

Medial meniscal injuries usually occur when an athlete is attempting to cut with a fixed foot. Damage results when rotational forces are applied to the knee while it is partially flexed with the foot on the ground. Medial meniscal injuries are commonly seen in sports such as soccer and football. Unfortunately, the medial meniscus is often damaged in conjunction with ligamentous injuries.

Lateral meniscal injuries are seen with less frequency than medial meniscal injuries. The lateral meniscus permits greater anatomic mobility and is thus less susceptible to tears. Damage to the lateral meniscus can occur when both rotational and compressive forces are applied to the knee while it is fully flexed with the foot fixed on the ground. These injuries can be seen in sports such as wrestling and in weightlifting when an athlete performs improper squatting.

### 4.1.1   Clinical Presentation

Patients usually present with intermittent medial, lateral, or diffuse knee pain and stiffness after a traumatic event. Some patients may not actually recall an inciting event. Others may report an audible "pop" during the injury. Patients often describe knee joint "clicking," "catching," "locking," or "giving way." Frequently, the knee becomes swollen within 24 hours.

### 4.1.2   Diagnosis

On physical exam, there is usually joint line tenderness. Medial joint line tenderness generally indicates damage to the medial meniscus. Likewise, tenderness over the lateral joint line usually implies lateral meniscal damage. Effusions are common.

During ROM testing, there frequently is a reduction in knee flexion and/or extension. Joint locking may occur as a result of displaced tears.

Special tests are useful for establishing a diagnosis. The anterior drawer test may be positive if there is ACL involvement. Other special tests include the McMurray test and the Apley compression test.

- *McMurray test:* Have the patient lie supine with the knee flexed. Palpate the joint line while applying a varus stress with the leg in internal rotation. Slowly extend the leg. The test is positive for a torn medial meniscus if a painful click is heard over the medial joint line. To test for lateral meniscal damage, apply a valgus stress with the leg in external rotation. The test is positive if a painful click is heard over the lateral joint line while extending the leg.
- *Apley compression test:* Also called the Apley grind test. Have the patient lie prone with the knee flexed to 90 degrees. Apply pressure downward on the heel while rotating the tibia on the femur. Pain over the medial joint line during external rotation indicates damage to the medial meniscus. Conversely, pain over the lateral joint line during internal rotation indicates injury to the lateral meniscus.

Diagnostic studies are helpful for confirming a diagnosis. Radiographs are usually normal. MRI has both high sensitivity and specificity for medial and/or lateral meniscal tears. Arthroscopy has the advantage of being both diagnostic and therapeutic.

### 4.1.3   Treatment

Patients should be treated conservatively in all but the most severe cases. Initial treatment consists of RICE, NSAIDs, and analgesics. Physical therapy is recommended for a partial-thickness tear with minimal displacement. Rehabilitation programs should incorporate ROM exercises, progressive strengthening beginning with isometric exercises and transitioning to closed kinetic chain exercises, and sports-specific agility training as the patient progresses. Arthroscopy should be considered in competitive athletes or patients who have failed conservative therapy. Most peripheral tears can be repaired since the outer one third of the meniscus is well vascularized. Any "locked" joint requires an urgent surgical evaluation.

### 4.1.4   Return to Play

Most patients return to their previous level of function. The exact timing of return to sports varies and depends on the severity of tear, treatment received, and specific rehabilitation protocol. In many cases, athletes can return to play as early as 2–3 weeks after arthroscopic partial meniscectomy. Other patients who require meniscal repair can return to play after 6–8 weeks.

# 5  Patellar Injuries

## 5.1  Patellofemoral Syndrome

Patellofemoral syndrome is a common disorder that is believed to be an overuse injury. Other names for this condition include "runner's knee" and "biker's knee." Patellofemoral syndrome is thought to occur as a consequence of poor biomechanics leading to abnormal tracking of the patella. Frequently, patellofemoral syndrome is incorrectly diagnosed as chondromalacia patella, which is a pathological diagnosis of patellar articular cartilage damage. Predisposing factors include increased exercise activity such as increased cycling or running distance.

### 5.1.1  Clinical Presentation

Patients often present with acute or insidious onset anterior knee pain that is worse with activity. Often the complaints are nonspecific such that the quality and location of the pain may vary. Usually the pain is related to overuse or change in intensity of the exercise. Activities that tend to worsen the pain are stair climbing, hill hiking, and squatting. Some patients report a painful catching sensation or a feeling of the knee "giving way."

### 5.1.2  Diagnosis

The physical exam is usually normal. There may be signs of patellar misalignment with abnormal tracking. Sometimes there is crepitation with patellar movement. Patellar compression may reproduce the discomfort. Occasionally there is tightness in the surrounding muscles, which can lead to patellar maltracking. Tenderness is often noted on the undersurface of the patella. This can be palpated by pressing down on the inferior portion of the patella with one hand and palpating the exposed undersurface of the superior patella with the other hand.

In addition, there may be an increased quadriceps (Q) angle. The Q angle is formed from the intersection of the long axes of the femur and tibia. Measure the Q angle by making a line from the anterior superior iliac spine to the midpoint of the patella, and a second line from the midpoint of the patella to the tibial tubercle. The "normal" Q angle varies from 10 to 20 degrees and is generally greater for females than for males. A Q angle >20 degrees may be abnormal. Other special tests include the patellar inhibition test.

- *Patellar inhibition test:* Also called the patella femoral grind test. Have the patient lie supine with the knee extended and relaxed. Apply stress to the superior aspect of the patella forcing it distally (Fig. 10.3). Next ask the patient to maximally contract the quadriceps. The test is positive if the patient is unwilling to do so or there is ensuing pain and crepitation on movement.

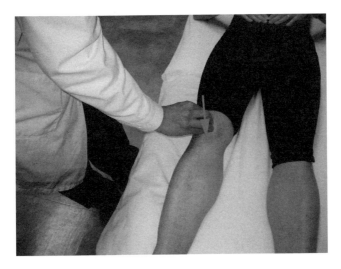

**Fig. 10.3** Patella inhibition test

Diagnostic studies are usually normal. Lateral plain films may show the presence of patella alta or patella baja. Sunrise or merchant's view permits better visualization of the patellofemoral articulation. Dynamic CAT scan is useful to assess patellar tacking in difficult cases. Arthroscopy is the procedure of choice for persistent symptoms despite conservative management.

### 5.1.3 Treatment

Most patients are successfully treated with conservative therapy. Initial treatment includes RICE, NSAIDs, analgesics, and activity modification. Most patients benefit from a trial of physical therapy. An optimal physical therapy regimen should incorporate quadriceps strengthening and stretching of the surrounding muscles. Most patients seem to better tolerate closed kinetic chain exercises. Some patients benefit from functional bracing. The most commonly used brace is a patellofemoral brace with a patellar cutout and lateral stabilizer. Other patients may benefit from McConnell taping to facilitate pain-free ROM. All patients should be encouraged to wear proper footwear.

Surgical treatment is reserved for patients who have failed conservative therapy lasting 6–12 months. A surgical consultation should be obtained for an obvious surgical lesion or recurrent disability.

### 5.1.4 Return to Play

Patients may return to play when symptoms allow and muscle strength has returned. It is recommended that athletes can return to previous activity when at least 80% of the strength of the uninjured knee has returned. This can be measured on isokinetic testing.

# 6 Tendinitis

## 6.1 Infrapatellar Tendonitis

Infrapatellar tendonitis is the most common cause of "jumper's knee." It is an overuse syndrome believed to be caused by repetitive stress on the patellar tendon during jumping. It is most frequently seen in sports that require extensive quadriceps loading during jumping, such as basketball, volleyball, and track and field. Overtraining and playing on hard surfaces are potential causative factors.

### 6.1.1 Clinical Presentation

Patients complain of an insidious onset of anterior knee pain usually localized to the inferior pole of the patella. Often the pain is described as "aching" and made worse with activity. Some patients may report a reduction in pain during the course of activity. Severe cases usually involve pain at rest.

### 6.1.2 Diagnosis

On physical exam, there is tenderness at the inferior pole of the patella and/or body of the patellar tendon. The remainder of the knee exam is usually normal. There may be associated tightness of the quadriceps or hamstrings compared with the uninjured side. Diagnostic imaging is usually normal. MRImay show signs of degeneration of the patellar tendon.

### 6.1.3 Treatment

Initial treatment involves RICE, NSAIDs, and the use of analgesics for pain control. Patients with mild to moderate disability are treated with activity modification and physical therapy. The goals of physical therapy are to restore pain-free ROM, strength, and flexibility. Some patients benefit from functional bracing. The most widely used brace is a patellofemoral brace with a patellar cutout and lateral stabilizer.

For patients with chronic, recurrent infrapatellar tendonitis, physical therapy that focuses on eccentric strengthening has been shown to be effective.

Patients with more severe disability might require relative rest for several weeks. A surgical consultation should be considered in patients with a complete tear or persistent disability despite conservative therapy.

### 6.1.4   Return to Play

Patients can return to play once they are asymptomatic. Athletes should be able to safely perform sport-specific activities.

## 7   Bursitis

### 7.1   *Iliotibial Band Syndrome*

Iliotibial band (ITB) syndrome is the most common cause of lateral knee pain among athletes. ITB syndrome is an overuse injury that results from an inflammation of the bursa as the ITB crosses the lateral femoral epicondyle. It is most common in runners and cyclists who require repetitive knee flexion and extension. Predisposing factors include increased running distance, especially downhill and hard-surface running.

### 7.1.1   Clinical Presentation

Patients usually present with an insidious onset of lateral knee pain worse with activity. Initially, the pain will resolve after activity; however, in severe cases, the pain will continue during walking. Occasionally, the pain will radiate below the knee or up into the lateral thigh. Some patients will complain of pain worse with ascending stairs or running downhill.

### 7.1.2   Diagnosis

On physical exam, there is tenderness over the lateral femoral epicondyle, located 2–4 cm above the lateral joint line. Pain is usually worse at approximately 30 degrees of knee flexion as the ITB passes over the lateral femoral epicondyle. During examination of gait, this pain may appear just after heel strike. Some patients will walk with the knee extended to avoid reproducing the pain. Special tests are useful for establishing a diagnosis.

- *Ober's test:* Used to assess the flexibility of the ITB. Have the patient lie on the uninvolved side. Stabilize the pelvis with one hand. Next abduct and extend the

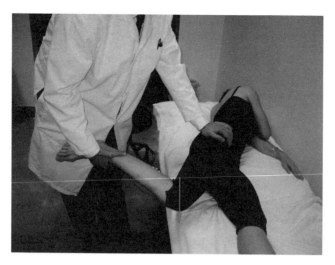

**Fig. 10.4** Ober's test

hip with the other hand. Once the hip is abducted, allow the hip to passively adduct toward the table (Fig. 10.4). A positive test results with resisted hip adduction.

- *Malacrea's test:* Have the patient lie on the uninvolved side. Next have the patient abduct the hip and extend the knee. Apply resistance to the leg while the patient flexes and extends the knee. A positive test occurs when there is reproduced pain in the area of the lateral femoral epicondyle.

Diagnostic imaging is usually normal unless there is an associated avulsion.

### 7.1.3 Treatment

Initial treatment involves RICE, NSAIDs, and analgesics for pain control. Most patients benefit from a trial of physical therapy. Physical therapy programs should incorporate active ITB stretching followed by strengthening of the hip muscles. Patients with no improvement after a few weeks may benefit from a steroid injection over the lateral femoral epicondyle. Surgery is rarely necessary. A surgical consultation should be considered in patients with recurrent disability despite conservative therapy. Prevention includes continuing ITB stretching and maintaining proper biomechanics during training.

### 7.1.4 Return to Play

Most patients can return to full activity once the pain has resolved and there is normal flexibility of the ITB. Ideally, the athlete should have regained full muscle strength in the hip and knee.

# 8  Apophysitis

## 8.1  Osgood-Schlatter Disease

Osgood-Schlatter apophysitis is a relatively common disorder classically seen in preadolescent boys who have undergone a growth spurt. Also called tibial tubercle apophysitis, Osgood-Schlatter disease results from repetitive quadriceps contraction through the patellar tendon at its insertion on the tibial tubercle. It is during preadolescence that the tibial tubercle is most susceptible to strain. Repeated traction can lead to microfractures at the apophysis.

### 8.1.1  Clinical Presentation

Patients typically complain of an insidious onset of pain at the site of the tibial tubercle after repetitive activities. The patient's symptoms are usually worse with running and jumping activities and improved with rest.

### 8.1.2  Diagnosis

On physical exam, there is tenderness over the tibial tubercle. This is sometimes associated with a soft tissue swelling. In some patients there may be tenderness over the patellar tendon. The remainder of the knee exam is usually normal. Patients may resist active knee flexion because of pain. Some patients have associated tightness in their hamstrings or quadriceps compared with the uninjured side.

Diagnostic imaging may show fragmentation of the tibial tubercle apophysis or the presence of an ossicle.

### 8.1.3  Treatment

Initial treatment includes RICE, NSAIDs, and the use of analgesics. Relative rest is recommended and to avoid activities that cause pain. Patients should be referred for physical therapy that includes a stretching and strengthening of the quadriceps and hamstring muscles. Ice is recommended as pain arises to avert recurrence of the disease. Some patients benefit from functional bracing. Surgery is rarely indicated. A surgical consultation should be considered in patients with recurrent disability not responding to conservative therapy.

### 8.1.4  Return to Play

Most cases are self-limiting. There is no contraindication to sports; however, patients will take longer to become asymptomatic if they do not rest.

# References

1. Barber FA, Sutker AN (1992) Iliotibial band syndrome. Sports Med. 14(2):144–148
2. Birrer RB, O'Connor FG (2004) Sports medicine for the primary care physician, 3rd edn. CRC Press, New York
3. Brindle T, Nyland J, Johnson DL (2001) The meniscus: review of basic principles with application to surgery and rehabilitation. J Athl Train 36(2):160–169
4. Cosgarea AJ, Jay PR (2001) Posterior cruciate ligament injuries: evaluation and management. J Am Acad Orthop Surg 9(5):297–307
5. Ferretti A (1986) Epidemiology of jumper's knee. Sports Med 3(4):289–295
6. Fredericson M, White JJ, Macmahon JM, Andriacchi TP (2002) Quantitative analysis of the relative effectiveness of 3 iliotibial band stretches. Arch Phys Med Rehabil 83(5):589–592
7. Griffin LY (1994) Sports medicine. John Wiley & Sons, New York
8. Juhn MS (1999) Patellofemoral pain syndrome: a review and guidelines for treatment. Am Fam Phys 60(7):2012–2022
9. Krause BL, Williams JP, Catterall A (1990) Natural history of Osgood-Schlatter disease. J Pediatr Orthop 10(1):65–68
10. Larson RL, Tailon M (1994) Anterior cruciate ligament insufficiency: principles of treatment. J Am Acad Orthop Surg 2(1):26–35
11. Lutz GE, Palmitier RA, Chao EYS, An KN (1993) Comparison of tibiofemoral joint forces during open and closed kinetic chain exercises. J Bone Joint Surg 75A:732–739
12. Lutz GE, Stuart MJ, Sim FH (1990) Rehabilitative techniques for athletes after reconstruction of the anterior cruciate ligament. Mayo Clin Proc 65:1322–1329
13. Reider B (1996) Medial collateral ligament injuries in athletes. Sports Med 21(2):147–156
14. Stuart MJ, Meglan DA, Lutz GE, Growney E, An KN (1996) Comparison of intersegmental tibiofemoral joint forces during various closed kinetic chain exercises. Am J Sports Med 24(6):792–799
15. Walsh WM (1990) Knee injuries. In: Taylor RB (ed) The team physician's handbook. Hanley & Belfus, Philadelphia

# Suggested Additional Reading

1. Birrer RB, O'Connor FG (2004) Sports medicine for the primary care physician, 3rd ed. CRC Press New York
2. Cooper G (2005) Pocket guide to musculoskeletal diagnosis. Humana Press, Totowa, NJ
3. Greene WB (2001) Essentials of musculoskeletal care, 2nd edn. American Academy of Orthopaedic Surgeons, Rosemont, IL
4. Griffin LY (1994) Sports medicine. John Wiley & Sons, New York
5. Hoppenfeld S (1976) Physical examination of the spine and extremities. Appleton-Century-Crofts, New York
6. Walsh WM (1990) Knee injuries. Taylor RB (ed) The team physician's handbook. Hanley & Belfus, Philadelphia

# Chapter 11
# Ankle and Foot Injuries

Aaron Levine and Dov Kolker

## 1  Anatomy

### *1.1  Bones*

The ankle mortise is composed of the medial malleolus (distal tibia), lateral malleolus (distal fibula), and talus. The bones of the foot include the seven tarsal bones (talus, calcaneus, navicular, cuboid, and three cuneiforms); five metatarsal bones; 14 phalanges with each digit having a proximal, middle, and distal phalange (the first toe has only a proximal and distal phalange); and two sesamoid bones located on the plantar aspect of the first metatarsal head. The foot can also be subdivided into three anatomical sections: the *forefoot* (composed of the metatarsals and phalanges), the *midfoot* (composed of the cuboid and cuneiforms), and the *hindfoot* (composed of the talus and calcaneus).

### *1.2  Ligaments*

The ankle joint is supported laterally by the lateral ligament which is composed of the anterior talofibular ligament (ATFL), the posterior talofibular ligament (PTFL), and the calcaneofibular ligament (CFL). Medial support is achieved by the medial ligament (deltoid ligament), which connects the medial malleolus to the talus, calcaneus, and navicular bones.

### *1.3  Muscles*

See Table 11.1.

J.E. Herrera and G. Cooper (eds.), *Essential Sports Medicine*,
doi: 10.1007/978-1-59745-414-8, © Humana Press 2008

**Table 11.1** Muscles of the ankle and foot

| Action | Muscles | Innervation |
|---|---|---|
| Ankle Dorsiflexors | Tibialis Anterior | Deep Peroneal n. |
| | Extensor Hallucis Longus | |
| | Extensor Digitorum Longus | |
| Ankle Plantarflexors | Tibialis Posterior | Tibial n. |
| | Gastrocnemius | |
| | Soleus | |
| | Flexor Hallucis Longus | |
| | Flexor Digitorum Longus | |
| | Peroneus Longus and Brevis | Superficial Peroneal n. |
| Ankle Inversion | Tibialis Anterior | Deep Peroneal n. |
| | Tibialis Posterior | Tibial n. |
| Ankle Eversion | Peroneus Longus and Brevis | Superficial Peroneal n. |
| | Peroneus Tertius | Deep Peroneal n. |
| Toe Flexion | Flexor Hallucis Longus and Brevis | Tibial n. |
| | Flexor Digitorum Longus and Brevis | |
| | Flexor Digiti Minimi Brevis | |
| | Interossei | |
| | Lumbricals | |
| Toe Extension | Extensor Digitorum Longus and Brevis | Deep Peroneal n. |
| | Extensor Digitorum Brevis | |
| | Lumbricals | Tibial n. |
| Toe Adduction | Adductor Hallucis | Tibial n. |
| | Plantar Interossei | |
| Toe Abduction | Abductor Hallucis | Tibial n. |
| | Abductor Digiti Minimi | |
| | Dorsal Interossei | |

## 1.4  Joints

See Table 11.2.

**Table 11.2** Foot and ankle joints

| Joint | Range of Motion |
|---|---|
| Ankle | Dorsiflexion: 10–20° |
| | Plantar Flexion: 45° |
| Subtalar (articulation of the talus and calcaneus) | Inversion: 5° |
| | Eversion: 5° |
| Forefoot (primarily at the midtarsal joint). | Adduction: 20° |
| | Abduction: 10° |
| First Metatarsophalangeal Joint | Flexion: 45° |
| | Extension: 80–90° |

## 1.5  Tarsal Tunnel

The tarsal tunnel is located between the posterior border of the medial malleolus and the Achilles tendon. The structures that run through this tunnel from an anterior to posterior direction are the Tibialis posterior tendon, the flexor Digitorum longus tendon, the posterior tibial Artery, the tibial Nerve, and the flexor Hallucis longus tendon. This can be remembered by the mnemonic "Tom, Dick, an' Harry."

## 2   Disorders of the Ankle

### 2.1   Ankle Sprains

Lateral ankle sprains are the most common form of ankle sprains and are caused by excessively inverting the ankle. This injury occurs in sports involving jumping (e.g., basketball, volleyball) when an athlete lands incorrectly and in sports involving abrupt direction changes (e.g., football, soccer). These ankle sprains involve partial or complete tears of the (ATFL, CFL, and/or PTFL, which are listed from most to least often injured. Damage to the medial ligamentous structures (i.e., deltoid ligament) occurs less commonly and is the result of an eversion injury. Associated fractures, such as a Maisonneuve fracture (proximal fibula fracture), and tibiofibular syndesmosis injuries should be ruled out.

#### 2.1.1   Clinical Presentation

Lateral ankle swelling and pain, particularly on the anterolateral aspect of the ankle, as well as pain with weight-bearing are common presenting symptoms of patients who have sustained lateral ankle sprains. The inability to weight bear should raise suspicion for an associated fracture. Patients reporting a pop at the time of injury or a feeling of ankle instability are more likely to have sustained a more severe sprain. Patients with a history of a prior ankle sprain/injury are at a higher risk for re-occurrence.

#### 2.1.2   Diagnosis

The diagnostic work-up is aimed at determining the type and severity of the injury in order to determine an appropriate treatment plan. Physical exam findings include swelling, ecchymosis, and tenderness to palpation at the site of the injury (i.e., over the injured ligamentous structure). The surrounding bony and tendinous structures, including the medial and lateral malleoli, should be examined for evidence of injury. Limitations of ROM and strength may be evident during the acute phase secondary to pain and should be monitored for return of function during the recovery phase. Special tests include the following.

- *Anterior drawer test:* This test evaluates the integrity of the ATFL. Place the foot in a neutral position and apply gentle anterior translation to the heel while using the other hand to stabilize the calf. Displacement >5 mm is considered to be a positive test. Compromise of the ATFL is also likely if there is increased excursion compared with the unaffected ankle or if there is a lack of a clear endpoint (Fig. 11.1).

- *Talar tilt test:* This test evaluates the integrity of the ATFL and CFL. Place an inversion stress on the talus. A difference in excursion of 10 degrees or more when comparing the affected and unaffected limbs is considered a positive test (Fig. 11.2).
- *External rotation test:* This test checks for injury to the tibiofibular syndesmosis. Apply an eversion stress to the injured ankle while in dorsiflexion. Pain at the distal portion of the tibiofibular junction is considered a positive test.

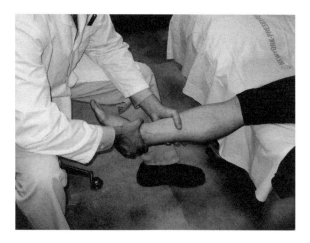

**Fig. 11.1**  Anterior drawer test

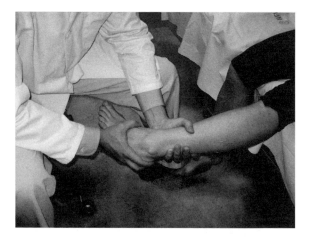

**Fig. 11.2**  Talar tilt test

Radiographic studies should include anteroposterior, lateral and mortise views and visualization of the fifth metatarsal is also important in order to exclude an avulsion fracture. Stress views (obtained while performing the anterior drawer and talar tilt testing) may be obtained if there is evidence of instability. If unsure of whether or not to obtain imaging studies, one can refer to the Ottawa ankle rules.

The Ottawa ankle rules are as follows: Obtain ankle x-rays if the patient has medial or lateral ankle pain and associated bony tenderness of the distal 6 cm of the posterior fibula or tibia. Obtain foot x-rays if there is midfoot pain and associated bony tenderness over the navicular bone or based of the fifth metatarsal. X-rays should also be obtained if the patient is unable to bear weight (Table 11.3).

### 2.1.3 Treatment

Initial management (1–3 days) involves RICE. Patients should keep off of the injured limb as much as possible, with or without the use of crutches. Compression can be achieved with an elastic bandage or compression stocking. NSAIDs and icing help with pain management and inflammation.

After the first few days following the injury, exercises to restore the ROM of the ankle, including Achilles tendon stretching, and to strengthen the ankle stabilizing muscles should be instituted. Weight-bearing exercises can be incorporated as the patient's pain permits. As the patient regains ankle strength and ROM, proprioceptive retraining, endurance exercises, and functional and sports-specific exercises should be added to the rehabilitation program. Additional ankle support through taping or bracing should be used initially and slowly phased out with time.

For patients with grade III injuries, a trial of conservative management may be instituted, but surgical consultation for consideration of surgical reconstruction may be necessary if nonsurgical treatment fails.

### 2.1.4 Return to Play

The severity of the injury as well as the demands of the sport should be considered when determining if an athlete is ready to return to sport. In general, if the patient's pain has resolved, full strength and ROM have been achieved, and functional/sports

**Table 11.3** Ankle sprain grading

| Grading | | |
| --- | --- | --- |
| Grade | Pathology | Findings on Stress Testing |
| Grade 1 | Partial ATFL tear<br>Intact CFL and PTFL | No ligament laxity |
| Grade 2 | Complete ATFL tear<br>Partial CFL tear | Ligament laxity<br>Firm endpoint |
| Grade 3 | Complete ATFL and CFL tear | Ligament laxity<br>No firm endpoint |

related exercises can be completed without pain, the athlete should be ready to return to sport. This may take only 1–2 weeks for less severe sprains but up to a couple of months for more severe sprains. Continued use of taping and bracing for a 3- to 6-month period is appropriate in those patients who sustained substantial ligamentous damage.

## 2.2 Achilles Tendinitis

This condition is due to inflammation and degeneration of the Achilles tendon (the common tendon for the gastrocnemius and soleus muscles). It is an overuse injury that occurs in such sports as running, especially when abruptly increasing mileage, and sports requiring repetitive jumping such as basketball, dancing, and volleyball. Other predisposing factors include overpronated feet, inadequate or new footwear, tight hamstrings and calf muscles, and anatomical foot disturbances (e.g., pes cavus).

### 2.2.1 Clinical Presentation

Patients present with pain in the posterior ankle along the course of the Achilles tendon. Symptoms usually are of gradual onset and occur primarily with activity and improve with rest. Pain severity varies considerably from patient to patient. Associated tendon swelling and stiffness are other common complaints.

### 2.2.2 Diagnosis

Physical exam may reveal pain when palpating the Achilles tendon, especially immediately proximal to its insertion on the calcaneus. The tendon should be palpated along its entire length in order to rule out tendon rupture. A painful nodule on the tendon may also be present. There may also be swelling in the region of the tendon. Patients presenting with chronic symptoms may have some associated plantarflexion weakness. Diagnostic imaging is usually not necessary. Ultrasound may be used to look for evidence of swelling and check for integrity of the tendon fibers. MRI can also be used if the diagnosis is uncertain.

### 2.2.3 Treatment

RICE should be instituted initially. NSAIDs can be used to address both the pain and inflammation. Ultrasound, massage therapy, and icing may also be useful for symptom management. A proper rehabilitation program should include Achilles tendon stretching and eccentric strengthening exercises and should be carried over into a comprehensive home exercise program. A heel raise/lift can be used to reduce strain on the tendon. Analyze the patient's footwear for proper fit, making sure it provides adequate rear foot support and prescribe orthotics if necessary. The use of corticosteroid injections is controversial as they may predispose a patient to developing tendon rupture. In general, they are not advisable. Surgical management involving adhesion release and débridement of degenerated tissue is rarely required and may serve as a last resort for those patients with chronic tendinitis that is refractory to conservative management.

### 2.2.4   Return to Play

Gradual return to play can begin once the patient's symptoms have resolved and the rehabilitation program has been completed, including sport-specific exercises. Proper footwear, with or without a heel lift, as well as continuing the home exercise program are also essential in order to prevent symptom recurrence.

## 2.3   *Achilles Tendon Rupture*

Patients may sustain a partial or complete rupture of the Achilles tendon. Partial ruptures are typically hard to distinguish from tendinitis and are often managed similarly, although partial ruptures tend to take longer to treat. This section focuses on complete tendon ruptures. The Achilles tendon is predisposed to rupture, typically within a few centimeters of the insertion onto the calcaneus, due to its poor vascularization in this region. A history of Achilles tendinitis, abrupt increases in training, participation in a new sport, and older age are predisposing factors. The inciting event usually involves sudden eccentric contraction of a dorsiflexed foot, which occurs in sports involving jumping and abrupt changes in speed (e.g., basketball, tennis).

### 2.3.1   Clinical Presentation

Presenting symptoms include acute onset of pain in the posterior ankle, swelling of the ankle and calf, an audible snap at the time of injury, and immediate plantarflexion weakness in the affected ankle. The patient may complain of significant difficulty walking.

### 2.3.2   Diagnosis

Physical exam often reveals a palpable gap in the tendon as well as a lump in the calf region due to retraction of the gastrocnemius and soleus muscles. Swelling in the lower portion of the calf is also common. Increased ankle dorsiflexion ROM as well as poor active ankle plantarflexion may be present. Thompson's test checks for the integrity of the Achilles tendon and is performed by squeezing the belly of the calf. If the tendon is ruptured, the foot should not plantarflex and the test is considered to be positive. MRI and ultrasound (US) can be used to evaluate the integrity of the tendon fibers but are not often needed since the diagnosis is often clear from the history and physical exam.

### 2.3.3 Treatment

Both conservative and surgical management options exist. Younger and more active patients are more likely to pursue surgical management to optimize function and performance. Patients who undergo surgical reattachment of the tendon are usually placed in a cast postoperatively, which is followed by gradual dorsiflexion of the ankle through serially casting or an adjustable brace (e.g., plantar flexion dial lock brace).

Nonsurgical management may also be appropriate in patients who are older, less active, or have complicating medical ailments making surgery more risky. Casting the ankle in a plantarflexed position for about 4 weeks is followed by gradual dorsiflexion by means of serially casting or an adjustable brace. After the bracing/casting is completed, a heel lift is used for a few months.

Once the cast is removed in either surgically or nonsurgically managed patients, a rehabilitation program should be implemented that includes soft tissue techniques, ROM exercises of the ankle, and gradual institution of strengthening exercises (eccentric strengthening program) with eventual progression to functional/sports-specific exercises.

### 2.3.4 Return to Play

For both the surgically and nonsurgically managed patients, a 6-month recovery period is typical prior to the patient being able to return to sport. This needs to be tailored to the individual patient based on successful completion of the rehabilitation program and the particular physical demands of the sport.

## 2.4 Retrocalcaneal Bursitis

Two bursae, one located between the Achilles tendon and the posterior aspect of the calcaneus and the other between the Achilles tendon and the skin, are susceptible to becoming inflamed and painful. In many patients, it may be difficult to distinguish bursitis from Achilles tendinitis, especially as they often occur simultaneously. Athletes, especially long distance runners, are quite susceptible to this injury due to overuse and repetitive pressure and trauma being placed on these bursae. Patients with a Haglund's deformity (enlarged posterosuperior lateral aspect of the calcaneus) or retrocalcaneal exostosis (bony proliferation of the posterior aspect of the calcaneus where the Achilles tendon inserts) are predisposed to this type of bursitis.

### 2.4.1   Clinical Presentation

Presenting symptoms include posterior heel pain and swelling that occur with activity. Inquire about a history of new footwear, sudden increases in training, and new athletic endeavors.

### 2.4.2   Diagnosis

Physical exam often reveals swelling, warmth, and tenderness to palpation of the posterior heel. Swelling and redness of the posterior heel (the "pump bump") may be present. As mentioned, it is often difficult to distinguish between bursitis and Achilles tendinitis, as symptoms and exam findings are very similar. One distinguishing exam finding is that patients with bursitis usually have pain when palpating the surrounding edges of the tendon, as opposed to patients with Achilles tendinitis who often have more tenderness along the tendon itself or near the calcaneal tendon insertion. Imaging studies are not usually necessary. If imaging is desired, MRI can be used to look at the bursae.

### 2.4.3   Treatment

Usually NSAIDs, relative rest from painful activities, and proper footwear are all that is required. A rehabilitation program that involves stretching of the Achilles tendon as well as a trial of modalities such as ultrasound and iontophoresis may also be useful. For those patients with persistent pain, a corticosteroid injection into the affected bursa can be used. Caution must be used when injecting in this area as it may predispose to weakening and even rupture of the Achilles tendon; therefore, more conservative measures are preferred. The affected bursa can be surgically excised if conservative measures fail.

### 2.4.4   Return to Play

The patient is ready to return to play once there has been symptom resolution and he or she is able to perform sports-specific and functional related exercises without pain.

## 2.5  *Plantar Fasciitis*

This condition is characterized by inflammation of the plantar fascia. The origin of the plantar fascia, the calcaneus, is the site most often affected. Activities such as running, prolonged standing or walking, dancing, and high-impact aerobics can cause repetitive microtrauma of the fascia leading to this condition. Other predisposing factors include a tight Achilles tendon, improper or new footwear, alterations in training intensity, pes planus, and pes cavus.

### 2.5.1  Clinical Presentation

Patients often present with complaints of pain in the heel and/or medial aspect of the foot. The pain is often worse during the first several steps after awakening in the morning, walking after prolonged sitting, and with activities that involve prolonged walking or running.

### 2.5.2  Diagnosis

Examine the patient's feet for predisposing anatomical disturbances such as pes planus/cavus as well as for over pronation of the foot during ambulation. Look for point tenderness at the proximal attachment of the fascia to the medial aspect of the calcaneus. Passive dorsiflexion of the great toe may elicit pain due to stretching of the plantar fascia. Diagnostic imaging studies are usually not required as the diagnosis is primarily based on the history and physical exam.

### 2.5.3  Treatment

Conservative management is very effective for most patients. The patient should avoid high impact activities that can aggravate symptoms (e.g., running, jumping). Stretching exercises focusing on the plantar fascia and Achilles tendon should be performed on a daily basis. Strengthening of the calf musculature is also important. Footwear adjustments may include shoes with proper support and flexibility, heel pads or cups, heel wedges, and arch supports. NSAIDs and modalities such as electrotherapy, massage therapy, and icing may help in pain control. A night splint that gently stretches the plantar fascia can be used. Consider local injection of corticosteroid into the fascia in patients with refractory symptoms. One must avoid injecting the corticosteroid into the superficial fat pad to prevent fat pad necrosis. A recent study has also suggested that botulinum toxin injections into the plantar fascia may be effective for this condition. When patients do not respond to conservative management, surgical referral for release of the aponeurosis from its origin may be considered.

### 2.5.4   Return to Play

Once the patient's symptoms have resolved and full painless ankle dorsiflexion has been achieved, gradual participation in sports is appropriate. This should be done while using proper footwear and foot supports as well as continuing to perform the stretching and strengthening exercises. Postsurgical patients can return to play in 3–4 months.

## 2.6   Flexor Hallucis Longus Tendinopathy/Injury

The flexor hallucis longus (FHL) is a great toe flexor and ankle plantar flexor. It originates from the distal portion of the fibula and interosseous membrane and inserts on the big toe at the base of the distal phalanx. Inflammation of the tendon typically occurs as it courses around the posterior aspect of the talus (between the medial and lateral tubercles) and into the tarsal tunnel. This injury occurs classically in ballet dancers presenting with pain in the medial aspect of the ankle but can occur in patients with poor fitting footwear or who participate in activities involving repetitive pushing off motions.

### 2.6.1   Clinical Presentation

The primary complaint is pain located along the course of the tendon, from the posteromedial aspect of the calcaneus to the great toe at the distal phalanx. The pain is usually activity related, occurring with activation and stretching of the FHL tendon.

### 2.6.2   Diagnosis

The diagnosis of this condition is based on history and physical exam findings, making imaging studies unnecessary in most cases. Pain is reproduced with palpation of the tendon along its course. Patients often report pain with active plantarflexion or passive dorsiflexion of the great toe.

### 2.6.3   Treatment

Conservative management is usually all that is required to treat this condition. NSAIDs used in conjunction with a stretching and strengthening program focusing on the FHL is the recommended treatment approach. Assess the patient's footwear as improper fitting shoes predispose patients to this condition. Technique during athletic endeavors should also be examined with corrections made as needed.

### 2.6.4   Return to Play

Gradual participation in sports is appropriate once the patient's symptoms have resolved and sports-specific exercises can be completed without pain. Use of proper footwear and technique is essential in preventing symptom recurrence.

## 2.7   Tibialis Anterior Tendinopathy

The tibialis anterior muscle acts to both invert and dorsiflex the ankle. The muscle originates at the lateral condyle and superior half of the lateral surface of the tibia and interosseous membrane. It inserts on the medial and inferior surfaces of the medial cuneiform and base of the first metatarsal. Inflammation of the tendon can occur as it runs under the superior retinaculum and is associated with overuse of the ankle dorsiflexors as well as with downhill running and overly tightened shoelaces.

### 2.7.1   Clinical Presentation

Patients often present with anterior ankle pain that is worse with movement of the ankle and better with rest. They may also complain that their foot slaps when they walk/run.

### 2.7.2   Diagnosis

Check for tenderness to palpation of the tibialis anterior tendon. Pain with active dorsiflexion and inversion or with passive plantar flexion of the ankle is common, with or without associated weakness. Imaging studies are not required.

### 2.7.3   Treatment

Treatment for this type of injury begins with reducing the pain and inflammation through a period of relative rest and NSAIDs. Once the patient is out of the acute phase, an eccentric strengthening program and ROM exercises of the ankle can be initiated with gradual inclusion of functional and sports-specific exercises as tolerated.

### 2.7.4   Return to Play

The patient is ready to return to play once there is symptom resolution and the rehabilitation program has been completed successfully, including the sports-specific training. This should be done gradually and the patient should continue the stretching and strengthening exercises.

## 2.8   Tibialis Posterior Tendon Injuries

The tibialis posterior tendon originates from the posterior tibia and fibula as well as the interosseous membrane and intermuscular septum. It passes posterior to the medial malleolus, where it makes a sharp direction change from a vertical to a horizontal direction and then inserts on the navicular tuberosity, cuboid bone, and middle three metatarsal bones. It acts to stabilize the medial aspect of the ankle as well as to plantarflex and invert the ankle. Tendon injury and inflammation usually occurs distal to the medial malleolus due to its relative poor blood supply after the tendon abruptly changes direction. Overuse is felt to be the culprit in patients with tendinitis, and may progress to tendon rupture when chronic inflammation and degenerative tendinosis occurs. Patients with a history of ankle inversion injuries tend to be more prone to this condition.

### 2.8.1   Clinical Manifestations

Patients complain of pain and swelling in the posteromedial aspect of the ankle and medial arch of the foot. Symptoms tend to be worse with prolonged walking or standing. Patients with tendon rupture may complain of ankle instability or weakness when attempting to push-off with the affected foot.

### 2.8.2   Diagnosis

Physical exam reveals posteromedial ankle pain with active ankle inversion. A valgus foot deformity as well as a flattened medial arch can be seen in patients with advanced tendinitis or tendon rupture. The "too many toes sign" may be observed due to the collapse of the medial arch. This sign refers to more toes being seen on the lateral aspect of the affected foot compared with the unaffected foot when viewing the patient from behind. Patients with a ruptured tibialis posterior tendon may also have an absence of the tibialis posterior tendon on palpation as well as associated plantar flexion and inversion weakness. If imaging studies are desired, MRI and ultrasound are helpful in evaluating the integrity of the tendon.

### 2.8.3   Treatment

Both surgical and nonsurgical management options are available. Tendinitis usually resolves with relative rest and NSAIDs followed by a rehabilitation program involving stretching, concentric and eccentric strengthening exercises, and sports-specific exercises. Fitting for orthotics may be appropriate in certain patients (e.g., patients with excessive foot pronation). Corticosteroid injections are not considered to be a safe treatment option by many due to the high risk of tendon rupture. Surgical débridement may be required in refractory cases. Patients with a ruptured tendon typically require surgical management, especially younger and more active patients.

### 2.8.4   Return to Play

For patients with tendinitis, return to play is appropriate once there is symptom resolution both at rest and with sports-related exercises. For patients who sustain a tendon rupture and undergo surgical repair, the surgeon will need to make the determination as to when the patient is ready to return to play as this varies considerably based on the severity of the tear and the type of surgical intervention used.

## 2.9   Peroneal Tendon Injuries

The peroneus longus and brevis muscles serve as everters and weak plantarflexors of the foot. The peroneus longus muscle originates from the lateral condyle of the tibia and head of the fibula and inserts on the base of the first metatarsal. The peroneus brevis muscle originates from the middle of the fibula and inserts on the base of the fifth metatarsal. Both tendinitis and tendon rupture can result from overuse injuries involving repetitive eversion (e.g., running on uneven surfaces, dancing, basketball, etc.) as well as from direct or indirect traumatic injuries such as lateral ankle sprains (i.e., inversion injuries).

### 2.9.1   Clinical Presentation

Patients complain of pain and swelling in the lateral ankle around the area of the lateral malleolus. Pain is often activity related. A feeling of ankle weakness and instability may indicate tendon rupture. Patients may also report a popping sensation in the lateral portion of the ankle.

### 2.9.2   Diagnosis

Swelling and tenderness on palpation along the course of the tendon(s) is present, especially behind the lateral malleolus. Provocative maneuvers include resisted ankle eversion and dorsiflexion as well as passive ankle inversion. Patients with tendon rupture often have ankle eversion weakness. MRI may be a useful diagnostic adjunct, especially if a tendon rupture is suspected based on the mechanism of injury, severity of symptoms, and physical exam findings. Evidence of tendinopathy (fluid/edema, scarring) or degenerative/traumatic tendon tears will show up on MRI.

### 2.9.3   Treatment

Conservative management is all that is required in most instances of peroneal tendinitis. This involves relative rest, NSAIDs, and icing. Once out of the acute phase, a stretching and strengthening program can be initiated. Strengthening of the peroneal muscles through resisted eversion is important. Taping or bracing may also be instituted initially to help protect the healing tendon(s).

In the case of tendon rupture, the patient should be referred for orthopedic evaluation for possible operative repair. Immobilization in plantarflexion for a 4- to 6-week period is a nonsurgical option for this type of injury.

### 2.9.4 Return to Play

Patients with peroneal tendinitis can gradually return to sports participation once the symptoms have resolved and successful completion of the rehabilitation program has been achieved. For patients with peroneal tendon ruptures, the determination of when the patient is ready to return to play is determined by the surgeon as the time course varies based on the degree of the tendon tear and the surgical approach that is used.

## 2.10 Sprain of the First Metatarsophalangeal Joint

Sprain of the first metatarsophalangeal (MP) joint is also commonly known as turf toe, as the use of artificial turf has increased the risk of this injury. It is caused by forced dorsiflexion (hyperextension) of the first MP joint, causing injury to the supporting capsule and ligamentous structures.

### 2.10.1 Clinical Presentation

Pain, swelling, and impaired ROM of the first MP joint is the most common complaint. The patient may also give a history of hyperextension of the first toe.

### 2.10.2 Diagnosis

Physical exam will often reveal a painful and swollen first toe with increased pain to palpation and ROM, which may also be reduced. Joint alignment and stability should be intact. X-rays may be useful to rule out fractures.

### 2.10.3 Treatment

Nonsurgical intervention is usually sufficient. RICE and decreased weight-bearing for the first few days are often adequate. Immobilization with taping and early institution of ROM exercises have been shown to be beneficial. The use of orthotics

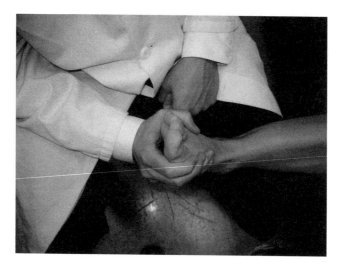

**Fig. 11.3** Tarsal compression test

and shoes with stiff soles can help in treating and preventing injury recurrence in these patients. Surgical referral for unstable and displaced intra-articular injuries is appropriate, although surgical intervention is rarely required (Table 11.4).

### 2.10.4 Return to Play

Once the pain and swelling have abated and sports-specific exercises can be completed without pain or a limp, return to play is appropriate. For grade III injuries, a period of 1–2 months may be required.

## 2.11 Morton's Neuroma

This condition involves swelling and inflammation of the interdigital nerve as it passes between the metatarsal heads. The nerve passing between the heads of the second and third and between the third and fourth metatarsals are the most commonly affected. Women are more often affected than men. Patients with poor footwear (e.g., narrow-fitting or tight-fitting footwear) or overly pronated feet are also more at risk for this condition.

### 2.11.1 Clinical Presentation

Forefoot pain on the plantar surface that is worse with weight-bearing is the primary complaint. Pain may radiate to the toes and there may be associated burning, numbness, or pins and needles.

**Table 11.4** MTP sprain grading

| Grading | | |
| --- | --- | --- |
| Grade | Pathology | Physical Exam Findings |
| Grade 1 | Capsular stretch injury | Minimal pain with weight bearing Mild MTP joint pain to palpation |
| Grade 2 | Partial tear of the plantar ligament complex | More severe pain with MTP palpation and with weight-bearing resulting in a limp |
| Grade 3 | Complete tear of the plantar ligament complex | Severe pain and swelling Inability to weight bear |

### 2.11.2 Diagnosis

There will often be localized tenderness to palpation of the space between the metatarsal heads or when compressing the metatarsal heads together (Fig. 11.3). An associated palpable click when compressing the affected web space may be evident. Radiographs are usually not needed except in patients with refractory symptoms.

### 2.11.3 Treatment

Pain control consists of NSAIDs and icing. Strengthening of the intrinsic muscles of the foot should be initiated as the patient's symptoms permit. Properly fitted and cushioned footwear, with or without the addition of metatarsal padding, can provide significant short- and long-term benefits. Local steroid injection can also help in reducing the patient's pain. Surgical excision of the neuroma is an option for those patients who fail conservative treatment, although there is a 5–10% recurrence rate.

### 2.11.4 Return to Play

Once the patient's symptoms have resolved and the ability to perform functional exercises asymptomatically has been achieved, the patient can gradually return to participation in sports. Proper footwear with adequate metatarsal padding will help prevent symptom recurrence.

## 2.12 Sinus Tarsi Syndrome

The sinus tarsi is an osseous canal bounded by the talus, calcaneus, talocalcaneonavicular joint, and posterior facet of the subtalar joint. The canal opens on the anterolateral aspect of the foot, just anterior to the lateral malleolus, and ends behind the sustentaculum tali. The canal contains vessels, subtalar ligaments, fat, and connective tissue. This condition is felt to be due to chronic synovitis of the subtalar joint secondary to ankle inversion injuries such as lateral ankle sprains or due to repetitive excessive foot pronation.

### 2.12.1  Clinical Presentation

Patients complain of pain in the area of the lateral opening of the sinus tarsi (i.e., the anterolateral aspect of the foot just anterior to the lateral malleolus). The symptoms are often worse with weight-bearing and exercise, especially when participating in sports that take place on uneven surfaces (e.g., outdoor walking/running). Complaints of foot and ankle stiffness and instability are also common.

### 2.12.2  Diagnosis

Localized pain to palpation over the lateral entrance to the sinus tarsi as well as restriction and pain with passive ROM of the subtalar joint are often found on physical exam. Placing an eversion stress on the subtalar joint may also reproduce the symptoms. Radiographs are not usually needed. Symptom resolution following injection of a short-acting local anesthetic is felt to be the best diagnostic test.

### 2.12.3  Treatment

The RICE principles should be used in the acute phase to address pain and inflammation. As symptoms improve, incorporation of a rehabilitation program involving gradual subtalar joint mobilization, progressive strength and proprioceptive training, and sports-specific exercises should be initiated. Corticosteroid injection into the sinus tarsi is an effective adjuvant to a comprehensive rehabilitation program. Surgical decompression is effective but rarely indicated.

### 2.12.4  Return to Play

Once the patient's symptoms have resolved and there has been successful completion of the rehabilitation program, including functional exercises, the patient can gradually begin participating in sports. Continuation of the stretching and strengthening exercises is important in preventing re-injury.

## 2.13  Metatarsalgia

This condition is characterized by forefoot pain located on the plantar surface of one or more metatarsal heads, primarily affecting the first two metatarsals. In athletes, training errors are the most common etiology, including rapid increases in training intensity and duration. Patients with overpronated feet are also more susceptible to this condition.

### 2.13.1 Clinical Presentation

Pain under the metatarsal head(s) is the typical complaint. This pain is initially only with weight-bearing but may progress to pain at rest. Patients may also complain of callus formation under the affected metatarsal head(s).

### 2.13.2 Diagnosis

The most common physical exam finding is pain with palpation of the first two metatarsal heads. Callus formation under the affected metatarsal heads may also be observed. The patient's gait should be examined for the presence of foot overpronation. Radiographs are not helpful in making the diagnosis but may be obtained to evaluate for underlying structural abnormalities such as metatarsal and toe malalignment.

### 2.13.3 Treatment

Conservative management is the mainstay of treatment. Initially, this involves relative rest and the use of NSAIDs. Metatarsal pads may also help relieve pressure from the metatarsal heads. Appropriate footwear with good arch supports is essential to treat and prevent symptom recurrence. Orthotics can be prescribed to correct excessive foot pronation. Rehabilitation also involves an individualized stretching and strengthening program to address improper biomechanics. Inclusion of sports-specific exercises and endurance training should gradually be incorporated.

### 2.13.4 Return to Play

Full participation in sports is appropriate once the patient's symptoms have resolved and he or she can carry out sport-specific exercises with minimal to no discomfort. Long-term use of prescribed orthotics is often necessary to prevent re-injury.

## 2.14 Heel Fat Pad Contusion

The fat pad over the heel of the foot serves as a shock absorber. It may be injured either by excessive forces being placed repetitively on the heel or due to a traumatic event such as a direct blow to the bottom of the heel. This type of injury occurs in sports players such as runners, long jumpers, and hurdlers, who have repetitive stresses placed on the heel. Footwear with poor heel cushioning also predisposes patients to this type of injury.

### 2.14.1 Clinical Presentation

Heel pain that occurs with weight-bearing and improves with rest is the most common complaint. Patients often give a history of participation in sports that places repetitive stress on the heels or occupations that involve prolonged walking or standing.

### 2.14.2 Diagnosis

Tenderness to palpation of the heel fat pad, especially over the weight-bearing portion of the calcaneus, is the most common finding. Bruising and atrophy of the fat pad may be observed. Plain films to rule out other pathology such as fractures and heel spurs are appropriate in refractory cases.

### 2.14.3 Treatment

RICE should be instituted initially, which should include the reduction of weight-bearing activities. Local steroid injections can be used in patients whose symptoms do not respond to activity modification and NSAIDs, but keep in mind the risk of causing steroid-induced fat necrosis when improper technique or multiple injections are used. A heel cup and properly cushioned footwear will also aid in healing and prevent recurrence.

### 2.14.4 Return to Play

Once symptoms have resolved and proper footwear has been acquired, the patient can return to play. Training errors such as increasing running mileage too quickly should be avoided.

## 2.15  Fractures

See Table 11.5.

**Table 11.5** Foot and ankle fractures

| Fracture type | Cause | Symptoms | Exam findings | Management | Return to play |
|---|---|---|---|---|---|
| Jones Fracture (Transverse fracture of diaphysis of 5th metatarsal) | Overuse injury or inversion of plantarflexed foot | Lateral foot pain with weight-bearing Swelling on lateral aspect of foot. | Tenderness to palpation, swelling and bruising in region of 5th metatarsal | Non-weight-bearing cast for 6 weeks vs. ORIF | Up to 20 weeks with conservative management  3–5 months if casted  8 weeks if patient had ORIF[a] |
| Avulsion Fracture of the 5th metatarsal | Ankle inversion injuries | Lateral foot pain with weight bearing | Tenderness to palpation and swelling over the proximal 5th metatarsal | Hard-soled shoe for 1 month | Typically in 3 to 4 weeks[a] |
| Dancer's Fracture (Spiral fracture of neck of 5th metatarsal) | Inversion injury: common in dancers due to missteps and fall from the Demi pointe position | Pain, swelling, bruising in lateral aspect of foot | Swelling, bruising and tenderness to palpation along 5th metatarsal | Non-displaced: relative rest and possible walking cast.  Displaced: 6–8 weeks in short leg cast but may require ORIF | The amount of time varies 6–52 weeks (average of 19 weeks)[b] |
| Lisfranc Fracture (Injury to the tarsometatarsal joints) | Axial loading on a plantarflexed foot | Pain and swelling in the dorsum of the midfoot | Pain with rotation of the forefoot while stabilizing the hindfoot | Non-displaced: 6–8 weeks non-weight-bearing and cast immobilization  Displaced: surgical stabilization | Typically 4–5 months after the injury[a] |
| March Fracture: (Stress Fracture: 2nd metatarsal and calcaneus most common | Increased activity level New activity (e.g., running, marching, sports that require repetitive jumping | Insidious onset of pain and swelling over area of fracture that is worse with ambulation | Fracture site point tenderness and/or swelling | Metatarsal: relative rest, protective footwear (e.g., stiff-soled shoe)  May require short leg cast.  Calcaneus: 6 weeks relative rest.heel cup or orthotic | In as little as 8 weeks: once asymptomatic and return of strength and ROM has been achieved |

(continued)

**Table 11.5** (continued)

| Fracture type | Cause | Symptoms | Exam findings | Management | Return to play |
|---|---|---|---|---|---|
| Pott's Fracture: Ankle fracture involving the lateral, medial, and/or posterior malleoli | Severe ankle inversion, eversion, or rotational injuries | Acute ankle pain Limited ability to weight-bear Swelling following inciting injury | Ankle swelling Focal tenderness at the affected malleolus Foot malalignment | Surgery: for displaced or unstable fractures: (Bimalleolar, lateral malleolar fx with deltoid ligament disruption, fracture-dislocations, trimalleolar) Conservative: Isolated non-displaced malleolar fractures treated with cast immobilization | Documentation of fracture healing, symmetric ROM and 85% of contralateral strength |
| Talar Dome Osteochondral Fractures | Associated with ankle sprains: inversion/eversion injuries | Ankle pain, swelling and stiffness. Symptoms persist despite treatment of ankle sprain | Impaired ROM Palpation tenderness of talar dome Effusion | Conservative management: immobilization, non-weight-bearing ORIF if conservative management fails | Varies based on the severity of the injury and the surgical approach that is used (determined by the surgeon) |
| Sesamoid Fractures | Stress fracture: common in tennis, basketball, dancing. Traumatic: jumping, forced dorsiflexion of the great toe | Forefoot pain with weight-bearing | Pain and swelling with palpation of the medial and/or lateral sesamoids | RICE, padding, possible short-leg cast or orthosis. May require non-weight-bearing for up to 6 weeks | Can begin 6 to 8 weeks (as symptoms permit)[c] |

[b]O'Malley MJ, Hamilton WG, Munyak J (1996) Fractures of the distal shaft of the fifth metatarsal. "Dancer's fracture" Am J Sports Med 24(2):240–243

[c]Gravlee J, Hatch L (6/28/2005) Sesamoid fractures of the foot. Up To Date

# References

1. Babcock M, Foster L, Pasquina P, Jabbari B (2005) Treatment of pain attributed to plantar fasciitis with botulinum toxin A: a short-term, randomized, placebo-controlled double-blind study. Am J Phys Med Rehabil 84(9):649–654
2. Bracker M (2001) The 5-minute sports medicine consult. Lippincott Williams & Wilkins, Philadelphia
3. Brukner P, Khan K (2002) Clinical sports medicine. McGraw-Hill, Sydney, Australia
4. Cuccurullo S (2004) Physical Medicine and Rehabilitation Board Review. Demos Medical Publishing, New York
5. Gravlee J, Hatch L (6/8/2005) Sesamoid fractures of the foot. Up To Date
6. Griffin L (2005) Essentials of musculoskeletal care, 3rd edn. American Academy of Orthopaedic Surgeons, Rosemont, IL
7. O'Malley MJ, Hamilton WG, Munyak J (1996) Fractures of the distal shaft of the fifth metatarsal. "Dancer's fracture." Am J Sports Med 24(2):240–243

# Chapter 12
# Hydration and Nutrition for the Athlete

**Earl L. Smith and Jeffrey I. Mechanick**

## 1  Introduction

Athletes must be aware of hydration and nutrition needs to support performance. Physicians function as educators for the child athlete through the Masters age group (> 50 years old) as well as athletes with a range of medical conditions, such as diabetes. In addition, physicians should know how treat casual as well as elite athletes, especially as recommendations for physical activity increase. Finally, the physician must be aware of the range of dietary supplements and nutraceuticals the athlete may be taking.

## 2  Hydration

There is a precise electrolyte balance between the intracellular and extracellular compartments, which maintains nerve and muscle function. Electrolyte balance is maintained by oral intake of electrolyte-containing substances, with excesses being renally excreted. The rate of absorption and excretion of fluids and electrolytes is hormonally mediated primarily by antidiuretic hormone (ADH), aldosterone, and parathyroid hormone (PTH). Variations from physiological levels may cause cardiac and neurological abnormalities.

Physicians need to be aware of both the risks of dehydration and overhydration, especially hyponatremia. The most important electrolyte is sodium, which is lost via perspiration. Low sodium levels may be further exacerbated by dilutional effects of overhydration. Potassium intake needs to be monitored as well, due to urinary losses and perspiration.

## 3  Dehydration

Heat, loss of water, and exercise are stressors that challenge normal homeostasis in athletes. Fluid replacement reduces the risk of heat-associated disorders and improves exercise performance. Greater than 2% loss of total body weight during

J.E. Herrera and G. Cooper (eds.), *Essential Sports Medicine*,
doi: 10.1007/978-1-59745-414-8, © Humana Press 2008

an exercise session can impair cardiovascular response. Maintenance of cardiac output allows skin perfusion and evaporative cooling via sweating. Fluids should be consumed in amounts equivalent to sweat loss. Received wisdom has suggested athletes need to replenish fluids by drinking a lot of water. Often, the athlete is told to "drink ahead of your thirst." However, in the past few years, the dangers of overhydration, especially in the nonelite athlete, has gained prominence. Overhydration with hypo-osmolar fluids has led to hyponatremia, and resulted in deaths of a handful of runners in the USA. One of the earliest high profile cases occurred in 2002, when a 28-year-old woman collapsed during the Boston Marathon and died of overhydration 2 days later. These risks are increasing as outdoors events such as iron man-style triathlons and ultramarathons grow in popularity. Long-distance and other endurance athletes need to be educated about the dangers of dehydration and low sodium.

## 3.1 Optimum Oral Rehydration During Exercise

The best method to determine rehydration needs are pre- and post-race weights. Weighing in before and after exercise can guide fluid requirements. Training should simulate potential race day ambient conditions: environment, terrain, duration, etc. The athlete should also consider insensate fluid losses associated with respiration when estimating hydration needs. By regularly checking pre- and post-training weights, the athlete will gradually learn to use subjective perceptions such as thirst, amount of perspiration and ambient conditions, and learn to estimate fluid need. This is analogous to the Borg perceived scale of exertion.

Daily water requirements for an average sized adult ( 70 kg) are around 2 liters plus exercise-related losses. Recommendations are mixed on the benefits of prehydrating with 1–2 (8 oz) glasses of water 2 hours prior and 1/2–1 glass immediately prior to exercise. Although this makes sense intuitively, most may be urinated out, depleting the body of needed sodium. Another 150–300 ml of water is required for every 15–20 minutes of exercise, but this is also variable. Postexercise, about 1–1.5 kg of water intake is required for every kg lost.

## 3.2 Diagnosis and Emergency Treatment of Dehydration

Physicians should be aware of and educate athletes as to warning symptoms (Table 12.1). Besides thirst, athletes may experience headaches similar to those of a hangover; visual field disturbances can occur in more severe cases. Clinical signs include hypotension, lightheadedness, and orthostatic hypotension, including fainting. Dehydration can lower blood pressure, and sitting in sauna or hot tub after an intense workout may further lower it through vasodilation and decreased venous return. The athlete should be aware of this phenomenon and instructed to

**Table 12.1** Maintaining fluid homeostasis: counseling athletes on hydration strategies

| Do | Don't |
| --- | --- |
| Replenish adequately fluid lost to perspiration, urination, and insensate losses. Learn to guide fluid requirements based on ambient conditions. | Don't overhydrate or drink too much plain water. Don't "drink ahead of your thirst." |
| If exercising >60 minutes, consume sports drinks containing electrolytes, especially sodium, and carbohydrate | Don't use sports drinks for workouts of <60 minutes |
| Check pre and postexercise weights | Do not eat solid/dry foods when dehydrated because water is required for digestion |
| Wear light-colored clothing. Adopt strategies to lower body temperature | Don't use too much sunscreen, which can impede cooling |

self-monitor for light-headedness. Left untreated, severe dehydration can result in delirium, loss of consciousness, seizures, and death.

Dehydration symptoms generally become noticeable after 2% of normal water volume has been lost. Initially, the athlete complains of thirst. Perspiration may decrease or cease and the athlete become flushed. Athletic performance may decrease up to 50%, as the athlete's endurance falls. Body temperature may rise and the athlete may become tachycardic and complain of fatigue. The symptoms become increasingly severe with greater water loss. The tachycardia is a compensation for the low blood pressure due to loss of plasma volume. As well, the hemoglobin/hematocrit may rise as the blood becomes concentrated. Flushing results from higher body temperature due to decreased perspiration.

At 5–6% water loss, somnolence, headache, nausea, and paresthesias may be reported. With 10–15% fluid loss, muscles may become spastic, skin may shrivel and wrinkle, vision may dim, urination will be greatly reduced and may become painful, and delirium may begin. Losses of >15% are usually fatal.

Early action may prevent worsening of symptoms. When dehydrated, a cool-off is essential to diminish unnecessary perspiration. This needs to be balanced with other training needs such as keeping the muscles warm to promote their recovery. If clinically dehydrated and replacement water is not available, the athlete should be counseled not to eat because water is required for digestion.

## 3.3 Prevention and Treatment of Dehydration

The first-line treatment is oral rehydration. Minor dehydration is best treated with oral rehydration with electrolyte-containing solutions such as sports drinks. Aqueous mixtures of salt, sugar, and water should be coadministered orally. The optimum concentration for efficient gastric emptying and osmotic balance is readily available in the form of commercial sports drinks. However, these sports drinks

**Table 12.2** Composition of repletion beverages

| Beverage | Sodium (mg/100 ml) | Potassium (mg/100 ml) | Carbohydrate (g/100 ml) | Comment |
|---|---|---|---|---|
| Gatorade® | 46 | 12.5 | 5.8 | |
| Skim milk | 51–54 | 146–167 | 5.4 | Varies with fat content, animal feed Protein = 3.3 g/100 ml |
| Chocolate milk | 80 | 140–170 | 10 | Protein = 3.2 g/100 ml |
| Pedialyte® | 104 | 78 | 5.0 | |
| Powerade® | 22 | 13 | 7.9 | |
| Amino Vital® | 4 | 15 | 1.7 | Amino acids = 308 mg/100 ml |
| Cola | 9–10 | Negligible | 11 | |
| Evian® | 0.5 | 0.1 | 0 | |
| New York City water | 0.6–5 | 0.04–0.26 | 0 | |
| Orange juice | 0 | 188 | 11 | |

may still not have enough sodium because they would be unpalatable if they had sodium levels equivalent to perspiration losses. Most carbonated beverages contain little or no sodium, affecting their osmotic balance and doing nothing to replenish the body. For these reasons, some athletes may require salt pills. Rehydration strategies can be simple: After a workout rehydration can be achieved with milk, which is rich in electrolytes. Sports drinks typically contain an appropriate concentration of carbohydrates ( 6%) to optimize gastric emptying and absorption in the gut. Emergency medical attention must be sought for more severe cases, e.g., fainting, loss of consciousness, altered mentation, or persistent nausea and vomiting. These symptoms demand intravenous rehydration. Rehydrating solutions, whether oral or IV, must contain electrolytes to replace those lost through perspiration or renal excretion. Generally only extended exercise, i.e., 60 minutes, requires the use of sports drinks. With less exertion, electrolytes and calories are adequately supplied by a balanced diet and an excess maybe be deleterious. Juices (real juices, not just sugary water and food color) or milk as well as sports drinks can nutritiously replenish lost electrolytes and replete muscle glycogen (Table 12.2).

## 3.4   Overhydration and Hyponatremia

Hyponatremia occurs in a substantial fraction of marathon runners and may be severe, especially in nonelite marathon runners. The use of NSAIDs may increase the risk of hyponatremia, so acetaminophen is a better choice of analgesic. Ultramarathon or iron man competitions may require the use of salt supplements. Attempts at water loading are futile because most of the preloaded water is urinated, further depleting the athlete of valuable salts. There have been recent reports of using triol glycerol as a water reservoir; however, this technique, although currently legal in international competition, has not yet been fully evaluated for safety.

## 3.5   Diagnosis and Emergency Management of Hyponatremia

Hyponatremia is simply an excess of water relative to sodium. In the hospitalized patient this is usually due to a prerenal state of an excess of ADH. However, in athletes, this may occur as a result of free water overconsumption without concurrent salt ingestion, coupled with sodium losses via perspiration. Hyponatremia is defined as a plasma sodium <135 mM, and may be further classified as mild (130–134 mM), moderate (126–129 mM), or severe (<126 mM). In severe cases of hyponatremia, cerebral edema and death can result. The extracellular fluid status is used to clinically divide hyponatremia into three categories to help to determine both the cause and treatment required. Hyponatremic patients' fluid status can be hypovolemic, euvolemic, or hypervolemic. Another distinction to make in evaluating hyponatremia is whether the onset was acute or chronic in nature. The confused or obtunded athlete is likely to be acute onset and hypervolemic. Physicians should rapidly assess the severity, risks, and potential need for emergency services. Hyponatremia should be in the differential diagnosis for athletes presenting with acute impairments. One scenario is when athletes present with symptoms suggestive of dehydration, e.g., muscle cramps, and are treated with intravenous fluids. Acute iatrogenic hypervolemic hyponatremia is fortunately rare but severe cases may result in respiratory distress and confusion. Treatment is with intubation, water restriction, and furosemide.

## 3.6   Symptoms of Hyponatremia

Runners most in danger of dehydration are not at the front of the race, but those at the back of the pack who spend more hours out in the heat. The elite athlete will finish a marathon before becoming too depleted, whereas the amateur athlete may require several hours to finish. Recent reviews have reported a fairly high incidence of hyponatremia in various marathon finishers. Participants should also be counseled regarding cooling strategies in lieu of drinking too much water. For example, some runners wear a white mesh cap containing ice cubes to reduce body temperature. Impediments to perspiration such as inappropriate clothing or too much sunscreen should be avoided. The athlete should consume sodium to replete losses. Good oral sources of sodium are low-fat salty foods, such as pretzels or salted crackers. Some runners may require salt pills. General guidelines suggest that marathon runners need 400–800 mg of sodium per hour during warm and hot weather conditions. The athlete should also be advised that urination may still continue even in a state of dehydration if hyponatremia develops as the body attempts to hemoconcentrate.

# 4    Nutrition for the Athlete

Athletes are preoccupied with body image, composition, and total mass. In weight-dependent sports such as running, weight loss may aid performance. Other sports such as boxing, football, or wrestling may require healthy weight gain. Athletes expect physicians to know the effects of nutrition on performance measures such as endurance, speed, or strength.

When dealing with athletes the first question physicians must ask is, "What type of exercise do they participate in?" For example, a body builder has very different goals and requirements than a marathon runner. Although total calories and protein are key issues to the strength athlete, carbohydrate and hydration aid endurance performance. Basic dietary prescriptions for health and fitness apply to athletes and nonathletes alike. They are given in the following.

1. Maintain a healthy body weight by adjusting food intake and exercise. This means an adequate supply of calories as well as the type of foods to optimize performance. Body mass index (BMI) from 18.5 to 25 may not be a desirable goal for some strength athletes, so physicians should be able to evaluate composition using other measures.
2. Eat less saturated fats, such as those fats found in animal products and tropical oils.
3. Eat sufficient protein. This should include a variety of nonanimal sources such as legumes, nuts, seeds, and grains.
4. In the absence of higher-quality research results, the athlete can generally follow the recommendations of the Institute of Medicine's Dietary Guidelines for Americans 2005, discussed in the following.

## 4.1    Requirements: Carbohydrate, Protein, Fluid, Vitamin, and Minerals

### 4.1.1    Carbohydrate

Adequate carbohydrate ingestion is required during and after exercise to replete/maintain glycogen stores. Carbohydrate contains 4 kCal/g; 6–8 g/kg of body mass are required daily. For a 70-kg (155-lb) athlete this is about 500 g/day or about 2000 carbohydrate calories of a 3000 calorie/day diet. Note this is significantly higher than for the sedentary. This is best consumed starches and fiber such as pasta, breads, or cereals containing whole grains. Timing is important: Ideally carbohydrates should be consumed within the first 20–40 minutes after exercise, to accelerate glycogen repletion. A good guideline is 1.5 carbohydrate/kg immediately after exercise followed by a second dose about 2 hours later, or about 100 g of carbohydrate for the 70-kg athlete. These can be easily accommodated in the daily requirement.

### 4.1.2 "Carbohydrate Loading"

Caution must be exercised to avoid ingesting too many calories—i.e., the nonelite athlete must be counseled that these are not weight loss supplements but in fact highly caloric. Conversely, the elite athlete and the overexerciser must be counseled on deterioration of performance if enough calories are not ingested. As well, some sports drinks are often very acidic and their high salt content makes the tooth enamel even more soluble than in plain water, so they may be erosive to teeth; they should be followed with a fresh water rinse when possible.

### 4.1.3 Protein Requirements for the Athlete

Guidelines for protein requirements are unresolved. Protein is the basic building material for muscle tissue and strength trainers need to consume more than nonexercisers. There is scant evidence that any particular profile of amino acids enhances endurance, strength, or hypertrophy. Commercial protein shakes, usually mostly whey, are becoming ever more popular. Their proteins may be partially hydrolyzed to enhance absorption. Amino acids such as glutamine, arginine, and branched chain amino acids (BCAAs) are used to enhance performance and muscle hypertrophy. However, it is not clear whether these preferentially enhance development and maintenance of type I versus type II muscle fibers. Maintaining a positive nitrogen balance enhances muscle growth and recovery. Even during rest breaks of a few days to weeks, high-protein diets have been shown to maintain muscle mass. There is no clear evidence that high-protein directly cause kidney problems when adequate hydration is maintained. Increased dietary protein may help athletes maintain muscle mass even during periods of rest from training. The recommended daily allowance of protein is about 0.8 g/kg per day. For endurance athletes, this is increased to 1.2–1.4 g/kg per day, and for strength athletes as much as 1.6–1.7 g/kg per day. For weight maintenance or loss, this can be up to 25% of calories, which is approximately 95 g of protein daily in a 1500 kCal diet, or 190 g of protein in a 3000 kCal diet. This is easily obtained with the typical American diet. Body-building magazines often recommend higher, such as 1–2 g of protein per pound of target body mass, although this can be difficult to attain without calorie overloading. The recommendations for serious strength athletes are about 0.6–0.8 g per pound of body weight, or about 95–125 g of protein/day for the 70-kg (155-lb) athlete and 128–164 g for one weighing 90 kg (200 lbs). Up to 0.1 g/kg of body mass consumed just prior

**Table 12.3** Protein Content of Common Foods

| | |
|---|---|
| 1 Large hard-boiled egg (50 g) | 6.3 g |
| 1 Cup (240 ml) skim milk | 3.4 g |
| 4 oz Yogurt | 6.5 g |
| 100 g Nonfat cottage cheese | 17.3 |

From Gabel KA (2006) Special nutritional concerns for the female athlete. Curr Sports Med Rep 5:187–191 to resistance training may be of some benefit. For the hypothetical 70-kg athlete, this would be 7 g of protein. Table 12.3 lists some common easily obtained foods containing about this amount of protein. Postexercise, protein intake may stimulate muscle repair, with some work showing prompt supplementation enhancing this effect. Protein supplementation during exercise has given mixed results on performance, and must be balanced with the known benefits of water, electrolyte, and carbohydrate supplementation; the utility of such supplementation beverages has been limited by palatability.

### 4.1.4 Fat

Fat intake should be about 20–35% of daily caloric intake. Very low fat diets can cause constipation, poor absorption of fat soluble vitamins, and essential fatty acid (EFA) deficiencies. After years of discussion in the specialist literature, the dangers of *trans*-fat has finally broken into the mainstream. Well known to raise HDL, they may also be harder to metabolize, even in the healthy athlete, slowing generation of energy. Good plant sources of EFAs include flaxseed, olive, soy, or canola oils, pumpkin and sunflower seeds, walnuts, and leafy vegetables. Good animal sources of EFAs include oily fish such as salmon and catfish, which are also rich in unsaturated ω-3 fatty acids such as EPA (eicosapentaenoic acid) and DHA (docosahexaenoic acid), as well as being good protein sources. There is no good evidence that branched chain fatty acids (BCFA) are superior to unbranched.

### 4.1.5 Dietary Supplements, Nutraceuticals, and Functional Foods

In the United States, any naturally occurring substance can be marketed with little or no oversight of nutritional claims. Table 12.4 lists some of the common herbal

**Table 12.4** Some dietary supplements and nutraceuticals encountered in sports medicine

| Nutraceutical | Proposed athletic benefit | Strength of evidence |
| --- | --- | --- |
| Androstenedione | Performance, body composition | D |
| Calcium | Increased bone density | A |
| Carnitine | Performance | C |
| Chondroitin sulfate | Osteoarthritis | B |
| Chromium | Weight loss (body composition) | D |
| Coenzyme-Q | Performance, antiaging | D |
| Creatine | Ergogenic | C |
| Dehydroepiandrosterone sulfate | Performance, body composition | D |
| Gingko biloba | Vasodilation | D |
| Glucosamine | Osteoarthritis | B |
| Glutamine | Performance | D |
| Ipriflavone | Bone density | B |
| Melatonin | Sleep | C |

*Strength of recommendation grades are assigned on the basis of the quality and consistency of the available evidence.

and other substances that have been proposed to enhance athletic activity, and summarizes the quality of evidence supporting or refuting their use.

A recent expert statement recommends that physicians should engage in frank discussion of supplements with athletes. Furthermore, only properly manufactured products should be used; physicians should advise against other products, and physicians should know the interactions with other foods or drugs. Physicians should also recommend against products with the potential to cause harm to the athlete. Other pitfalls athletes must be aware of are, comparable to those of the sedentary, maintaining a healthy diet away from home, such as in restaurants or institutional settings such as residence halls.

In the absence of better firm nutrition information, the Institute of Medicine's (IOM's) Dietary Guidelines for Americans 2005 are the definitive authority. These guidelines were also adopted by the American Heart Association in 2006. The guidelines recommend an overall healthy diet, aiming for a healthy body weight (body mass index between 18.5 and 24.9 kg/m$^2$), and a desirable lipid profile. The IOM also does not make any recommendations about any supplements or nutraceuticals but instead suggests plant-derived foods rich in antioxidant nutrients, such as fruits, vegetables, whole grains, and vegetable oils.

IOM also recommends a healthy diet whole-grain, high-fiber foods; consuming fish at least twice a week; limiting intake of saturated fat to <7% of energy, *trans* fat to <1% of energy, and cholesterol to <300 mg/day; minimizing added sugars and salt; and consuming alcohol in moderation. Guidelines for fat intake are now more restrictive. The goals can be achieved by choosing lean meats and vegetables, selecting fat-free (skim) or low-fat (1% fat) dairy products, and minimizing the use of hydrogenated fats used in commercial food preparation. They also recommend consumption of oily fish high in EPA and DHA, while specifying the avoidance of fish which may be high in mercury such as shark or mackerel.

## 5  The Female Athlete

The female athlete triad is defined as the presence of anorexia nervosa, amenorrhea, and osteoporosis. This typically occurs in the peripubertal female when oral intake is not sufficient to meet needs in the setting of psychosocial and environmental stressors, and vigorous athletic training. Even when the female athlete does not meet all the criteria for this triad, athletic performance may be compromised with overtraining and undernutrition.

## 6  The Master's Category

Our society is aging and the baby boomer generation shows historically unprecedented levels of recreational and sporting activity. Most sporting events include Masters categories for patients older than 50, 60, 70, or even 90. These athletes are especially vulnerable to the risks of dehydration, but on the other hand are especially receptive to educational messages on nutrition and hydration. Generally, aging is associated with decreased lean mass, increased fat mass, and often decreased recuperative powers. In the absence of other health conditions, e.g., heart disease, osteoporosis, or anemia, Master's athletes are generally counseled similarly to other adults, taking into account medical conditions such as heart disease, decreased renal and liver metabolism, and the lower resting metabolic rate. There is a paucity of research related to Master's athletes, and this represents an expanding field of interest.

## 7  The Pediatric Athlete

Pediatric athletes are at risk of overtraining. Children are at risk of not maintaining adequate nutrition for optimum performance. Their caloric needs are constantly changing. One of the first symptoms of inadequate nutrition is complaints of declining performance. If performance gains are adequate, the pediatric athlete is generally counseled similarly to the adult population after the age of 2.

## 8  The Diabetic Athlete

Diabetes can be especially challenging as physical activity requires an increased carbohydrate intake. The diabetic must be counseled to check blood sugar levels more often and adjust caloric intake accordingly, because muscle contraction can increase insulin action and glucose uptake. Rapid absorbing carbohydrates in the form of juice or hard candies should be on hand in case of hypoglycemia. As well, the patient's insulin should be readily available. In the event of hyperglycemia (FS > 300), this is best treated by insulin and rest, not exercise.

## References

1. Almond CS, Shin AY, Fortescue EB, et al. (2005) Hyponatremia among runners in the Boston Marathon. N Engl J Med 352:1550–1556
2. Ayus JC, Arieff A, Moritz ML (2005) Hyponatremia in marathon runners. N Engl J Med 353:427–428
3. Bar-Or O (2001) Nutritional considerations for the child athlete. Can J Appl Physiol 26 Suppl: S186–191
4. Beals KA, Hill AK (2006) The prevalence of disordered eating, menstrual dysfunction, and low bone mineral density among US collegiate athletes. Int J Sport Nutr Exerc Metab 16:1–23
5. Campbell WW, Geik RA (2004) Nutritional considerations for the older athlete. Nutrition 20:603–608
6. Coyle EF (2004) Fluid and fuel intake during exercise. J Sports Sci 22:39–55
7. Dallam GM, Jonas S, Miller TK (2005) Medical considerations in triathlon competition: recommendations for triathlon organisers, competitors and coaches. Sports Med 35:143–161
8. De La Torre DM, Snell BJ (2005) Use of the preparticipation physical exam in screening for the female athlete triad among high school athletes. J Sch Nurs 21:340–345

9. De Souza MJ, Hontscharuk R, Olmsted M, Kerr G, Williams NI (2006) Drive for thinness score is a proxy indicator of energy deficiency in exercising women. Appetite 88(4):974–975
10. De Souza MJ, Alleyne J, Vescovi JD, Williams NI, VanHeest JL, Warren MP (2007) Correction of misinterpretations and misrepresentations of the female athlete triad. Br J Sports Med 41:58–59
11. DiPietro L, Stachenfeld NS (2006) The myth of the female athlete triad. Br J Sports Med 40:490–493
12. Ebell MH, Siwek J, Weiss BD, et al. (2004) Strength of recommendation taxonomy (SORT): a patient-centered approach to grading evidence in the medical literature. J Am Board Fam Pract 17:59–67
13. Forsberg S, Lock J (2006) The relationship between perfectionism, eating disorders and athletes. A review. Minerva Pediatr 58:525–536
14. Gabel KA (2006) Special nutritional concerns for the female athlete. Curr Sports Med Rep 5:187–191
15. Goudie AM, Tunstall-Pedoe DS, Kerins M (2005) Altered mental status after a marathon. N Engl J Med 352:1613–1614
16. Griffin LY (2005) Emergency preparedness: things to consider before the game starts. J Boine Joint Surg 87A:894–902
17. Halperin ML, Kamel KS, Sterns R (2005) Hyponatremia in marathon runners. N Engl J Med 353:427–428; author reply 427–428
18. Herbold NH, Frates SE (2000) Update of nutrition guidelines for the teen: trends and concerns. Curr Opin Pediatr 12:303–309
19. Hew TD (2005) Women hydrate more than men during a marathon race: hyponatremia in the Houston marathon: a report on 60 cases. Clin J Sport Med 15:148–153.
20. Hew TD, Chorley JN, Cianca JC, Divine JG (2003) The incidence, risk factors, and clinical manifestations of hyponatremia in marathon runners. Clin J Sport Med 13:41–47
21. Horswill CA (1998) Effective fluid replacement. Int J Sport Nutr 8:175–195
22. Inder WJ, Swanney MP, Donald RA, Prickett TC, Hellemans J (1998) The effect of glycerol and desmopressin on exercise performance and hydration in triathletes. Med Sci Sports Exerc 30:1263–1269
23. Institute of Medicine (2006) Dietary reference intakes: the essential guide to nutrient requirements. The National Academies, Washington, DC
24. Jensen J (2004) Nutritional concerns in the diabetic athlete. Curr Sports Med Rep 3:192–197
25. Jeukendrup AE, Jentjens RL, Moseley L (2005) Nutritional considerations in triathlon. Sports Med 35:163–181
26. Kratz A, Siegel AJ, Verbalis JG, et al. (2005) Sodium status of collapsed marathon runners. Arch Pathol Lab Med 129:227–230
27. Lawrence ME, Kirby DF (2002) Nutrition and sports supplements: fact or fiction. J Clin Gastroenterol 35:299–306
28. Lerand SJ, Williams JF (2006) The female athlete triad. Pediatr Rev 27:e12–3
29. Levenhagen DK, Carr C, Carlson MG, Maron DJ, Borel MJ, Flakoll PJ (2002) Postexercise protein intake enhances whole-body and leg protein accretion in humans. Med Sci Sports Exerc 34:828–837
30. Levenhagen DK, Gresham JD, Carlson MG, Maron DJ, Borel MJ, Flakoll PJ (2001) Postexercise nutrient intake timing in humans is critical to recovery of leg glucose and protein homeostasis. Am J Physiol Endocrinol Metab 280:E982–993
31. Levine BD, Thompson PD (2005) Marathon maladies. N Engl J Med 352:1516–1518
32. Lisle DK, Trojian TH (2006) Managing the athlete with type 1 diabetes. Curr Sports Med Rep 5:93–98
33. Loucks AB, Nattiv A (2005) Essay: the female athlete triad. Lancet 366(Suppl 1):S49–50
34. Loucks AB, Stachenfeld NS, DiPietro L (2006) The female athlete triad: do female athletes need to take special care to avoid low energy availability? Med Sci Sports Exerc 38:1694–1700
35. Maharam LG, Bauman PA, Kalman D, Skolnik H, Perle SM (1999) Masters athletes: factors affecting performance. Sports Med 28:273–285

36. McCaffree J (2006) Managing the diabetic athlete. J Am Diet Assoc 106:1161–1162
37. Mechanick JI, Brett EM (2005) Nutrition and the chronically critically ill patient. Curr Opin Clin Nutr Metab Care 8:33–39
38. Mechanick JI (2005) The rational use of dietary supplements and nutraceuticals in clinical medicine. Mt Sinai J Med 72:161–165
39. Mechanick JI, Brett EM, Chatusmer AB, Dickey RA, Wallach S (2003) American Association of Clinical Endocrinologists Medical Guidelines for the Clinical Use of Dietary Supplements and Nutraceuticals. Endocrine Pract 9:417–470
40. Miller KK (2003) Mechanisms by which nutritional disorders cause reduced bone mass in adults. J Womens Health (Larchmt) 12:145–150
41. Montain SJ, Cheuvront SN, Sawka MN (2006) Exercise associated hyponatraemia: quantitative analysis to understand the aetiology. Br J Sports Med 40:98–105; discussion 98–105
42. Noakes T (2003) Fluid replacement during marathon running. Clin J Sport Med 13:309–318
43. Orchard JW, Fricker PA, White SL, Burke LM, Healey DJ (2006) The use and misuse of performance-enhancing substances in sport. Med J Aust 184:132–136
44. Peate WF (2005) Hyponatremia in marathon runners. N Engl J Med 353:427–428; author reply 427–428
45. Reid SA, Speedy DB, Thompson JM, et al. (2004) Study of hematological and biochemical parameters in runners completing a standard marathon. Clin J Sport Med 14:344–353
46. Rock CL (1991) Nutrition of the older athlete. Clin Sports Med 10:445–457
47. Saunders MJ, Kane MD, Todd MK (2004) Effects of a carbohydrate-protein beverage on cycling endurance and muscle damage. Med Sci Sports Exerc 36:1233–1238
48. Sherman RT, Thompson RA (2006) Practical use of the International Olympic Committee Medical Commission Position Stand on the Female Athlete Triad: a case example. Int J Eat Disord 39:193–201
49. Shirreffs SM, Armstrong LE, Cheuvront SN (2004) Fluid and electrolyte needs for preparation and recovery from training and competition. J Sports Sci 22:57–63
50. Speedy DB, Thompson JM, Rodgers I, Collins M, Sharwood K, Noakes TD (2002) Oral salt supplementation during ultradistance exercise. Clin J Sport Med 12:279–284
51. Speedy DB, Noakes TD, Schneider C (2001) Exercise-associated hyponatremia: a review. Emerg Med (Fremantle) 13:17–27
52. Stoddard DW (2004) Fluid replacement during marathon running. Clin J Sport Med 14:248; author reply 248–250
53. Von Duvillard SP, Braun WA, Markofski M, Beneke R, Leithauser R (2004) Fluids and hydration in prolonged endurance performance. Nutrition 20:651–656
54. Warren MP, Goodman LR (2003) Exercise-induced endocrine pathologies. J Endocrinol Invest 26:873–878
55. Wharam PC, Speedy DB, Noakes TD, Thompson JM, Reid SA, Holtzhausen LM (2006) NSAID use increases the risk of developing hyponatremia during an Ironman triathlon. Med Sci Sports Exerc 38:618–22

## Selected Websites

1. http://www.nyc.gov/html/dep/pdf/wsstat03c.pdf. vol. 2007
2. http://www.nal.usda.gov/fnic/foodcomp/search/. vol. 2007
3. http://www.healthyeatingclub.com/info/books-phds/books/foodfacts/html/data/data5b.html. vol. 2007
4. http://www.health.gov/dietaryguidelines/dga2005/document/html/appendixB.htm. vol. 2007
5. http://www.supplementshack.com. vol. 2007
6. http://www.mineralwaters.org. vol. 2007

# Chapter 13
# Banned and Approved Substances

**Daniel Leung, Joseph E. Herrera, and Lisa Bartoli**

Physicians who participate in the treatment of competitive athletes must have a clear understanding of the anti-doping regulations that exist. The consequences for violating these regulations can be severe for athletes. In addition, medical practitioners should be aware that they can be found guilty of anti-doping violations as well. These include prescribing, trafficking, or otherwise assisting athletes in taking banned substances.

There are governing bodies such as the World Anti-Doping Agency (WADA), International Olympic Committee (IOC), and sport specific governing bodies that create regulations regarding suspensions, and exemptions of athletes that use banned substances. When in doubt, check with the appropriate governing body to get a full list of banned and approved substances. These regulations are constantly evolving as does new technology and methods of doping. Medical practitioners and athletes should both be aware of these constant changes. For instance, caffeine was removed from the prohibited list in 2004 as was dermatological glucocorticosteroid preparations in 2005. Following is a sample list of prohibited substances adopted from WADA guidelines. It is always good practice to review doping and testing protocols with athletes prior to each competition.

In some cases certain banned substance may be permitted when a medical need arises, and a therapeutic exemption is given. One common example of this is seen in athletes who are asthmatic. Beta agonists, such as albuterol, are banned in nonasthmatic athletes due to the stimulant effect that they may give once administered. With a therapeutic exemption asthmatic athletes are permitted to use this medication. When obtaining a therapeutic exemption it is recommended that the athlete, medical team, and/or coach keeps multiple copies and always retains receipt of approval from the sports-governing body. It is not unusual that the athlete is asked to provide the appropriate proof before, during, and after competition.

J.E. Herrera and G. Cooper (eds.), *Essential Sports Medicine*,
doi: 10.1007/978-1-59745-414-8, © Humana Press 2008

**Sample List of Prohibited Substances (Adopted from WADA Guidelines)**

Substances Prohibited at All Times (In and Out of Competition)

1. Anabolic agents
2. Hormone and related substances:
   Examples include but are not limited to erythropoietin (EPO), growth hormone (hGH), insulin-like growth factors (ie: IGF-1), mechano growth factors (MGFs), gonadotrophins (LH, hCG)-prohibited in males only, insulin, and corticotrophins
3. Beta-2-agonists (requires therapeutic use exemption)
   All beta-2 agonists, including their D- and L- isomers, are prohibited. Formoterol, salbutamol, salmeterol, and terbutaline by inhalation are permitted with a therapeutic use exemption. However a concentration of salbutamol >1000 ng/ml will be considered an adverse analytical finding, unless the athlete can prove the abnormal result was a consequence of the therapeutic inhalation.
4. Agents with anti-estrogenic activity:
   Aromatase inhibitors including, selective estrogen receptor modulators (SERMs) and other anti-estrogenic substances including, but not limited to, clomiphene, cyclofenil, and fulvestrant.
5. Diuretics and other masking agents:
   Diuretics, which include acetazolamide, amiloride, bumetanide, canrenone, chlorthalidone, ethacrynic acid, furosemide, indapamide, metolazone, spironolactone, thiazides, triamterene, and other substances with similar chemical structure and biological effects (drospirenone is not prohibited).

**Methods Prohibited In Competition and Out of Competition**

1. Enhancement of oxygen transfer:
   Blood doping, and the use of products such as to perfluorochemicals, Efaproxiral (RSR13), and modified hemoglobin products are banned
2. Chemical and physical manipulation:
   Substitution and/or alteration of urine or blood products are illegal.
3. Gene doping

## Substances Prohibited In Competition (These Are in Addition to Those Prohibited at All Times)

1. Stimulants:
   Include the following (both D- and L- isomers):

The following is a short list of some of the stimulants that are banned. Refer to WADA or governing association of the specific sport for a full listing of medications. The banned medications include the following: Adrafinil, adrenaline, amphetamine, amphetaminil, bromantan, carphedon, cathine, cocaine, dimethylamphetamine, ephedrine, ethamivan, fenethylline, fenfluramine, mefenorex, mephentermine, mesocarb, methylephedrine, methylphenidate, modafinil, pemoline, penteterazol, phendimetrazine, phenmetrazine, phenpromethamine, phentermine, prolintane, propylhexedrine, selegiline, sibutramine, strychnine.

Adrenaline in conjunction with local anesthetic agents are not prohibited (ie: ophthalmic and nasal preparations). Cathine is prohibited if urine concentrations exceed 5 μg/mL. Ephedrine and methylephedrine are prohibited if urine concentrations >10 μg/mL.

Stimulants that are not prohibited, but are on the 2006 Monitoring Program In-Competition include bupropion, caffeine, phenylephrine, phenylpropanolamine, pipradrol, pseudoephedrine, and synephrine. Please confirm with the sport-specific governing body regarding banned status of the medication.

2. Narcotics (use caution when prescribing pain meds):
   Buprenorphine, dextromoramide, diamorphine (heroin), fentanyl and its derivatives, hydromorphone, methadone, morphine, oxycodone, oxymorphone, pentazocine, pethidine
3. Cannabinoids
4. Glucocorticosteroids (may require Therapeutic Use Exemption):
   All glucocorticosteroids are prohibited when administered orally, rectally, intravenously, or intramuscularly. Their use requires a Therapeutic Use Exemption approval. Topical use preparations when use dermatological, aural/otic, nasal, buccal cavity, and ophthalmological disorders are not prohibited and do not require any form of Therapeutic Use Exemption.

## Substances Prohibited in Particular Sports

1. Alcohol:
Alcohol (ethanol) is prohibited in-competition only in the following sports. Detection is made via blood or breath samples with maximal threshold in parenthesis.

| Sport | Alcohol level (g/L) | Sport | Alcohol level (g/L) |
|-------|---------------------|-------|---------------------|
| Aeronautic | (0.20) | Karate | (0.10) |
| Archery | (0.10) | Modern pentathlon for disciplines | |
| Automobile | (0.10) | involving shooting | (0.10) |
| Billiards | (0.20) | Motorcycling | (0.10) |
| Boules | (0.10) | Powerboating | (0.30) |

2. Beta-blockers:
Beta-blockers are prohibited in-competition for the following sports:

Aeronautics, archery (as well as out-of-competition), automobiles, billiards, bobsleigh, bridge, chess, curling, gymnastics, motorcycling, modern pentathlon for disciplines involving shooting, nine pin bowling, sailing for match race helms only, shooting, skiing/snowboarding in ski jumping, freestyle aerials/half-pipe and snowboard half-pipe/big air, and wrestling.

## Specified Substances-Substances that are Particularly Susceptible to Unintentional Anti-Doping Violations Because of General Availability in Medicinal Products

1. All inhaled beta-2 agonists (except clenbuterol)
2. Probenecid
3. Certain stimulants
4. All glucocorticosteroids
5. Alcohol
6. All beta-blockers

# References

1. Blue JG, Lombardo JA (1999) Steroids and steroid-like compounds. Clin Sports Med 18:667–689
2. Burke L (2003) Sports supplements and sports foods. In: Hargreaves M, Hawley J (eds) Physiological bases of sports performance. McGraw-Hill, Sydney, Australia
3. Geyer H, Parr MK, Mareck U et al. (2004) Analysis of non-hormonal nutritional supplements for anabolic androgenic steroids-results of the international IOC study. Int J Sports Med 25:124–129
4. Green GA, Catlin DH, Starcevic B (2001) Analysis of over-the-counter dietary supplements. Clin J Sport Med 11:254–259
5. International Olympic Committee (2000) Olympic Movement Anti-Doping Code. IOC, Lausanne, www.olympics.org
6. Magkos F, Kavouras S (2004) Caffeine and ephedrine: physiological, metabolic and performance-enhancing effects. Sports Med 34:871–889
7. Orchard JW, Fricker PA et al. (2006) The use and misuse of performance-enhancing substances in sport. MJA 184 (3):132–136
8. Spriet LL (1995) Caffeine and performance. Int J sports Nutr 5:S84–S89
9. Striegel H et al. (2005) The World Anti-Doping Code 2003: consequences for physicians associated with elite athletes. Int J Sports Med 26:238–243
10. World Anti-Doping Agency (WADA) (2006) The 2006 Prohibited List International Standard. WADA, Montreal, www.wada-ama.org
11. World Anti-Doping Agency (WADA) (2003) World Anti-Doping Code. WADA, Montreal, www.wada-ama.org
12. World Anti-Doping Agency (WADA) (2004) Therapeutic Use Exemptions. Abbreviated process. WADA, Montreal, www.wada-ama.org

# Index

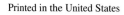

Printed in the United States